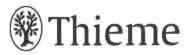

PRP and Microneedling in Aesthetic Medicine

Amelia K. Hausauer, MD
Fellowship-Trained Cosmetic Dermatologist
Director of Dermatology
Aesthetx
Campbell, California, USA

Derek H. Jones, MD
Cosmetic Fellowship Director
American Society for Dermatologic Surgery
Medical Director
Skin Care and Laser Physicians of Beverly Hills
Los Angeles, California, USA

62 illustrations

Thieme
New York • Stuttgart • Delhi • Rio de Janeiro

Executive Editor: Stephan Konnry
Managing Editor: Nikole Y. Connors
Director, Editorial Services: Mary Jo Casey
Production Editor: Torsten Scheihagen
International Production Director: Andreas Schabert
Editorial Director: Sue Hodgson
International Marketing Director: Fiona Henderson
International Sales Director: Louisa Turrell
Director of Institutional Sales: Adam Bernacki
Senior Vice President and Chief Operating Officer:
    Sarah Vanderbilt
President: Brian D. Scanlan

Library of Congress Cataloging-in-Publication Data

Names: Hausauer, Amelia K., editor. | Jones, Derek, 1965- editor.
Title: PRP and microneedling in aesthetic medicine
    / [edited by] Amelia K. Hausauer, Derek H. Jones.
Description: First edition. | New York : Thieme, [2019] |
    Includes bibliographical references. |
Identifiers: LCCN 2019001716 (print) | LCCN 2019005428
    (ebook) | ISBN 9781626239050 (e-book) | ISBN
    9781626239043 (print) | ISBN 9781626239050 (eISBN)
Subjects: | MESH: Cosmetic Techniques | Head–surgery |
    Platelet-Rich Plasma | Injections, Intradermal
Classification: LCC RD119 (ebook) | LCC RD119 (print) |
    NLM WE 700 | DDC 617.9/5–dc23
LC record available at https://lccn.loc.gov/2019001716

Copyright © 2019 by Thieme Medical Publishers, Inc.
Thieme Publishers New York
333 Seventh Avenue, New York, NY 10001 USA
+1 800 782 3488, customerservice@thieme.com

Thieme Publishers Stuttgart
Rüdigerstrasse 14, 70469 Stuttgart, Germany
+49 [0]711 8931 421, customerservice@thieme.de

Thieme Publishers Delhi
A-12, Second Floor, Sector-2, Noida-201301
Uttar Pradesh, India
+91 120 45 566 00, customerservice@thieme.in

Thieme Publishers Rio de Janeiro, Thieme Publicações Ltda.
Edifício Rodolpho de Paoli, 25º andar
Av. Nilo Peçanha, 50 – Sala 2508,
Rio de Janeiro 20020-906 Brasil
+55 21 3172-2297 / +55 21 3172-1896
www.thiemerevinter.com.br

Cover design: Thieme Publishing Group
Typesetting by DiTech Process Solutions

Printed in Germany   8 7 6 5 4
by Beltz Grafische Betriebe

ISBN 978-1- 2623-904-3

Also available as an e-book:
eISBN 978-1-62623-905-0

Important note: Medicine is an ever-changing science undergoing continual development. Research and clinical experience are continually expanding our knowledge, in particular our knowledge of proper treatment and drug therapy. Insofar as this book mentions any dosage or application, readers may rest assured that the authors, editors, and publishers have made every effort to ensure that such references are in accordance with **the state of knowledge at the time of production of the book.**

Nevertheless, this does not involve, imply, or express any guarantee or responsibility on the part of the publishers in respect to any dosage instructions and forms of applications stated in the book. **Every user is requested to examine carefully** the manufacturers' leaflets accompanying each drug and to check, if necessary in consultation with a physician or specialist, whether the dosage schedules mentioned therein or the contraindications stated by the manufacturers differ from the statements made in the present book. Such examination is particularly important with drugs that are either rarely used or have been newly released on the market. Every dosage schedule or every form of application used is entirely at the user's own risk and responsibility. The authors and publishers request every user to report to the publishers any discrepancies or inaccuracies noticed. If errors in this work are found after publication, errata will be posted at www.thieme.com on the product description page.

Some of the product names, patents, and registered designs referred to in this book are in fact registered trademarks or proprietary names even though specific reference to this fact is not always made in the text. Therefore, the appearance of a name without designation as proprietary is not to be construed as a representation by the publisher that it is in the public domain.

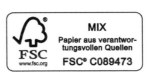

To our loving families without whom this text would not have been possible. They endured our efforts and were de facto part of the team. Thank you for being supportive always.

Contents

Menu of Accompanying Videos

Products and Devices used in the videos are provider and preparatory system specific and may vary. There is no standard protocol; rather, the demonstration videos provide good examples by experts who have performed many cases with excellent outcomes.

Preface

The body has an extraordinary capacity to heal itself, a potential that we tap into daily but still do not fully understand the extent or **ways to best direct**. With the advent of bone marrow and solid organ transplant came a new field of medicine: regenerative medicine. Coined in 1992 by William Haseltine, PhD, founder of the Human Genome Sciences, this term refers to a specialty dedicated to the creation of "living, functional tissue to repair and replace [those] lost due to age, disease, damage, or congenital defects.[i] Rejuvenation is one branch of regeneration with the goal of **stimulating the body's own repair mechanisms to heal previously altered or damaged cells.[ii]** Essentially, how to enhance self-healing. Platelet rich plasma (PRP) and microneedling are two increasingly popular modalities intended to harness these abilities. They can be used independently or in combination to capitalize on the release of growth factors critical for not only wound healing but also extracellular matrix synthesis and remodeling as well as hair cycling.

First described in the 1990s,[iii] *medical* microneedling and concentrated platelet therapies have taken off with new articles available nearly monthly. Given this growing interest, we sought to create a reference for key literature published to date; practical considerations important when appraising different delivery methods; as well as data or, when unavailable, experience-driven protocols to optimize patient care. The Food and Drug Administration (FDA)-clearance and regulation of these devices is a continually changing landscape. None are directly approved for rejuvenation, scar revision, or hair restoration but are often used in these off-label (in the United States) indications. This text does not directly review current legislature, since it may be country and state specific. Instead, our purpose is to appraise both the basic and clinical science supporting use of PRP and microneedling in aesthetic medicine in order to identify best practices and drive future research.

Mayo clinic website:

Regenerative medicine is a game-changing area of medicine with the potential to fully heal damaged tissues and organs, offering solutions and hope for people who have conditions that today are beyond repair.

Regenerative medicine itself isn't new — the first bone marrow and solid-organ transplants were done decades ago. But advances in developmental and cell biology, immunology, and other fields have unlocked new opportunities to refine existing regenerative therapies and develop novel ones.

The Center for Regenerative Medicine takes three interrelated approaches:

- **Rejuvenation.** Rejuvenation means boosting the body's natural ability to heal itself. Though after a cut your skin heals within a few days, other organs don't repair themselves as readily.
But cells in the body once thought to be no longer able to divide (terminally differentiated) — including the highly specialized cells constituting the heart, lungs and nerves — have been shown to be able to remodel and possess some ability to self-heal. Teams within the center are studying how to enhance self-healing processes.

- **Replacement.** Replacement involves using healthy cells, tissues or organs from a living or deceased donor to replace damaged ones. Organ transplants, such as heart and liver transplants, are good examples.
The center aims to expand opportunities for transplants by finding ways to overcome the ongoing donor shortage, the need for immunosuppression and challenges with organ rejection.

- **Regeneration.** Regeneration involves delivering specific types of cells or cell products to diseased tissues or organs, where they will ultimately restore tissue and organ function. This can be done through cell-based therapy or by using cell products, such as growth factors. Bone marrow transplants are an example.

Regenerative medicine holds the promise of definitive, affordable health care solutions that heal the body from within.

Wikipedia:

Regenerative medicine deals with the "process of replacing, engineering or regenerating human cells, tissues or organs to restore or establish normal function." This field holds the promise of engineering damaged tissues and organs by stimulating the body's own repair mechanisms to functionally heal previously irreparable tissues or organs.

NIH

https://report.nih.gov/NIHfactsheets/ViewFactSheet.aspx?csid=62

Regenerative medicine is the process of creating living, functional tissues to repair or replace tissue or organ function lost due to age, disease, damage, or congenital defects. This field holds the promise of regenerating damaged tissues and organs in the body by stimulating previously irreparable organs to heal themselves. Regenerative medicine also empowers scientists to grow tissues and organs in the laboratory and safely implant them when the body cannot heal itself. Importantly, regenerative medicine has the potential to solve the problem of the shortage of organs available through donation compared to the number of patients that require life-saving organ transplantation.

i. https://www.healthcanal.com/public-health-safety/ 50621-um-leads-in-the-field-of-regenerative-me- dicine-moving-from-treatments-to-cures-2.html
ii. Orentreich DS, Orentreich N. Subcutaneous incisionless (subcision) surgery for the correction of depressed scars and wrinkles. Dermatologic surgery : official publication for American Society for Dermatologic Surgery [et al] 1995;21:543-9.
iii. Camirand A, Doucet J. Needle dermabrasion. Aesthetic Plast Surg 1997;21:48-51.

https://www.karger.com/Article/FullText/477353

Contributors

Brian J. Abittan, MD
Icahn School of Medicine
Mount Sinai
New York, New York

Tina S. Alster, MD
Director
Washington Institute of Dermatologic Laser Surgery
Clinical Professor of Dermatology
Georgetown University Medical Center
Washington, DC

Matthias Aust, PhD
Associate Professor
Private Practice for Plastic Surgery
Bad Woerishofen, Germany

R. Lawrence Berkowitz, MD
Diplomate American Board of Plastic Surgery
Aesthetx Surgery Center
Campbell, California

Jeanette M. Black, MD
Dermatologist
Skin Care and Laser Physicians of Beverly Hills
Los Angeles, California

Chatchadaporn Chunharas, MD
Cosmetic Laser Dermatology
San Diego, California

DiAnne S. Davis, MD, MS
Chief Resident Physician
Department of Dermatology
University of Oklahoma HSC
Oklahoma City, Oklahoma

Lisa M. Donofrio, MD
Assistant Clinical Professor
Department of Dermatology
Yale University School of Medicine
Madison, Connecticut

Gary Goldenberg, MD
Goldenberg Dermatology
Assistant Clinical Professor
Department of Dermatology
Icahn School of Medicine at Mount Sinai
New York, New York

Mitchel P. Goldman, MD
Medical Director
Cosmetic Laser Dermatology
San Diego, California

Aditya K. Gupta, MD, PhD
Department of Medicine
University of Toronto
School of Medicine
Toronto, Ontario, Canada
Mediprobe Research Inc.
London, Ontario, Canada

Peter W. Hashim, MD, MHS
Department of Dermatology
Icahn School of Medicine at Mount Sinai
New York, New York

Amelia K. Hausauer, MD
Fellowship-Trained Cosmetic Dermatologist
Director of Dermatology
Aesthetx
Campbell, California, USA

Derek H. Jones, MD
Cosmetic Fellowship Director
American Society for Dermatologic Surgery
Medical Director
Skin Care and Laser Physicians of
    Beverly Hills
Los Angeles, California, USA

Tatjana Pavicic, MD, PhD
Doctor
Private Practice for Dermatology and
    Aesthetics
Munich, Germany

Brenda L. Pellicane, MD
Washington Institute of Dermatologic
    Laser Surgery
Washington, DC

Jeffrey A. Rapaport, MD
Medical Director
Cosmetic Skin and Surgery Center
Englewood Cliffs, New Jersey

Naissan O. Wesley, MD
Dermatologist/Dermatologic Surgeron
Clinical Instructor
Department of Medicine
Division of Dermatology
David Geffen School of Medicine
University of California Los Angeles
Skin Care and Laser Physicians of Beverly Hills
Los Angeles, California

Douglas C. Wu, MD, PhD
Cosmetic Laser Dermatology
San Diego, California

Sarah G. Versteeg, MSc
Mediprobe Research Inc.
London, Ontario, Canada

Kamakshi Zeidler, MD
Aesthetx Surgery Center
Campbell, California

Part I

Platelet-Rich Plasma Principles and Practices

1

Platelet-Rich Plasma: Mechanism and Practical Considerations

Brian J. Abittan and Gary Goldenberg

Abstract

Platelet-rich plasma (PRP) has many potential uses in Dermatology. Autologous PRP is retrieved from a patient's whole blood and spun in a centrifuge to yield a final product of plasma with high concentrations of platelets. These platelets then activate and release key growth factors that initiate signaling cascades, ultimately maximizing tissue repair and rejuvenation. Many systems are available to obtain PRP. It is critical to appraise these systems objectively and consider all the factors that are needed for both the patient and setting in which PRP will be used.

Keywords: platelet-rich plasma (PRP), mechanism of action, systems appraisal, preparations, practical considerations

Key Points

- Platelet-rich plasma has multiple uses in dermatology.
- Complete understanding of the mechanisms of action is unknown. However, stimulation of growth factors triggered contained within platelets plays a key role.
- There are multiple delivery systems available on the market.
- It is the key to evaluate and understand the advantages and disadvantages of these systems.

1.1 Introduction

There has been increasing interest in the utilization of autologous platelet-rich plasma (PRP) for the management of various clinical entities. First described for use in tissue repair[1] and hemostasis,[2] PRP has been applied more recently to a multitude of medical and cosmetic conditions, including in orthopedics,[3] dentistry,[4] plastic surgery,[5] and dermatology,[6] as seen in ▶ Table 1.1. Several studies seek to evaluate the effectiveness of PRP for androgenic alopecia, skin rejuvenation, and hair transplantation surgery.

Table 1.1 PRP Uses in dermatology and other medical fields

PRP uses In dermatology[6,8]	PRP uses in other medical fields[3,5,7,9,10,11]
<ul><li>Androgenic alopecia</li><li>Scar revision</li><li>Acne scarring</li><li>Skin rejuvenation</li><li>Dermal augmentation</li><li>Striae distensae</li><li>Skin aging</li><li>Wrinkles</li><li>Melasma and dyspigmentation</li><li>Hair transplantation surgery</li><li>Periocular circles</li></ul>	<ul><li>Tendinopathy</li><li>Muscle injury</li><li>Bone remodeling</li><li>Osteoarthritis</li><li>Bone grafts</li><li>Sinus lifts</li><li>Fat transfers</li><li>Breast augmentation</li><li>Wound healing</li><li>Dental bone rejuvenation</li><li>Periodontal wound healing</li><li>Severe dry eye syndrome</li><li>Ocular surface syndrome post LASIK surgery</li></ul>

Abbreviation: PRP, platelet-rich plasma.

However, very few randomized controlled trials exist and as such the literature is lacking qualitatively.[7] That being said, with PRP's increasing prevalence in aesthetic practices, it is crucial to understand what PRP is and its mechanism of action. The PRP preparation process must be thoroughly understood to effectively distinguish between various available systems (▶ Table 1.1).[3,5,6,7,8,9,10,11]

1.2 Definition of Platelet-Rich Plasma

PRP is an autologous preparation of plasma with high concentrations of platelets derived from whole blood.[12] Normal platelet levels in blood range from 150,000 to 400,000 platelets/µl or 150 to 400×10^9/L. The working definition of PRP today is plasma containing greater than 1,000,000 platelets/µl, based on studies showing bone and soft tissue healing enhancement at this level.[13] Today, most PRP preparations have a concentration that is 4 to 8 times higher than that of peripheral blood,[9] depending on the preparation system.

Studies have shown that the growth factors contained within PRP increase linearly with elevated platelet concentrations.[14] Giusti et al noted the induction of angiogenesis in endothelial cells was optimized with a platelet concentration of 1,500,000 platelets/µl. Additionally, it was also determined that extremely high concentrations of platelets actually decreased angiogenesis.[15] This negative correlation was also seen in studies revealing an inhibitory impact on bone regeneration with extremely high platelet concentrations.[16]

Using an autologous preparation of PRP affords multiple advantages. It decreases concern of immunogenic reactions and makes disease transmission unlikely.[17]

Thus, the procedure is quite safe, well tolerated, and has minimal side effects.

PRP is differentiated from recombinant growth factors in that they are physiological, derived intrinsically from the humans rather than animal models or cell medium, and thereby contain "pure" growth factors. Additionally, they are delivered via a clot, which is a natural delivery system in humans. Recombinant growth factors are extracted from an external system, usually from other animals, and delivered via synthetic carriers.[13] PRP contains both leukocytes, which are catabolic and proinflammatory, along with platelets and plasma, which produce anabolic functions within the body. It is crucial that these seemingly opposing functions are balanced appropriately, allowing each to accomplish its purpose. Even small changes in the levels of these growth factors could create an imbalance, yielding an increase in inflammation and or pain.[10] It is hypothesized that maintaining an unadulterated balance of anabolic and catabolic functions helps maintain the optimal environment for tissue healing and growth.[9]

1.3 Basic Science behind PRP and Proposed Mechanism of Action for PRP

The mechanisms of PRP are not fully understood. However, it is believed that the platelets release signaling proteins, including a multitude of growth factors, chemokines, and cytokines, that result in the promotion of cell proliferation and differentiation.[4,12,18,19] Platelets are known to contain more than 20 growth factors[20] inside their α-granules, which are released upon activation in order to deliver the signaling molecules into surrounding tissue. ▶ Table 1.2 lists important growth factors, such as platelet-derived growth factor (PDGF), transforming growth factor (TGF), epidermal growth factor (EGF), vascular endothelial growth factor (VEGF), insulin-like growth factor (IDGF), and interleukin 1 (IL-1) (▶ Table 1.2).[14,18,19,21,22,23,24,25]

Table 1.2 PRP growth factors and their primary functions[14,2223,24,25]

Growth factor	Actions
PDGFαα, PDGF αβ, PDGF ββ	• Chemotactic for fibroblasts, macrophages, and neutrophils • Mitogenic for fibroblasts, smooth muscle cells, endothelial cells, mesenchymal cells, and osteoblasts • Promotes synthesis of collagen and other proteins, regulates collagenase secretion
TGF-β1, TGF-β2, TGF-α	• Promotes angiogenesis • Regulation of cell proliferation, differentiation, and apoptosis • Chemotactic for fibroblasts, keratinocytes, and macrophages • Mitogenic for fibroblasts, smooth muscle cells • Inhibits endothelial cells, keratinocyte, lymphocyte, and macrophage proliferation • Regulates matrix proteins production (collagen, proteoglycans, fibronectin, and matrix degrading proteins) • Proliferation of undifferentiated mesenchymal cells
VEGF	• Stimulates angiogenesis and vessel permeability • Chemotactic and mitogenic for endothelial cells
FGF-2, FGF-9	• Involved in tissue regeneration • Stimulates growth and differentiation of mesenchymal cell, chondrocytes, osteoblasts
EGF	• Heavily involved in regulating cell proliferation, differentiation, and survival • Stimulates angiogenesis • Mitogenic for fibroblasts, endothelial cells, mesenchymal cells, and keratinocytes • Promotes endothelial chemotaxis • Regulates collagenase secretion
IGF-1	• Regulates cell metabolism • Stimulates proliferation and differentiation in osteoblasts (bone formation) • Chemotactic for fibroblasts • Stimulates protein synthesis

Table 1.2 continued

Growth factor	Actions
CTGF	• Promotes angiogenesis, chondral regeneration, fibrosis, and platelet adhesion

Abbreviations: CTGF, connective tissue growth factor; EGF, epidermal growth factor; FGF, fibroblast growth factor; IGF, Insulin-like growth factor; PDGF, platelet-derived growth factor; PRP, platelet-rich plasma; TGF, transforming growth factor; VEGF, vascular endothelial growth factor.

The platelets in PRP secrete most of their growth factors within an hour of activation,[22] with residual factors being released for up to 7 days.[13] The mechanisms by which PRP likely achieves efficacy have been well described in other fields of medicine: orthopedics, surgery, dentistry, and wound healing. PRP increases the release of cytokines, which then bind to the surface of cellular transmembrane receptors, causing intracellular signaling. This effectuates change at the microscopic level including angiogenesis, collagen synthesis, extracellular matrix production, and decreased apoptosis, mimicking the mechanisms needed for dermatologic uses.[3,26]

In dermatology, the proposed mechanism of PRP varies based on its location of use. As noted, growth factors released by platelets in PRP may stimulate different targets based on specific areas treated.

1.3.1 Mechanism of Action for PRP Effects on Hair Growth

PRP stimulates hair growth via many mechanisms, but one important pathway is anagen-associated angiogenesis.[12,27] Numerous treatments for hair loss have been aimed at increasing angiogenesis and improving blood flow to the hair follicle unit.[4] Secretion of vascular endothelial growth factor (VEGF) is largely responsible for the anagen-associated angiogenesis and has also been shown to augment growth of dermal structures.[28,29] Beyond VEGF, the α-granules in PRP release increased levels of PDGF and, platelet-derived endothelial growth factor. These factors are hypothesized to work on the stem cells of hair follicles and stimulate neovascularization.[30] As such, PRP has been used to effectively treat male and female hair loss (▶ Fig. 1.1).[19] Improved circulation in the structures immediately surrounding hair follicles indicates a clear mechanism for improved hair growth.[20] Similarly, subcutaneous injections of PRP have improved the survival of skin grafts, likely by a similar mechanism of increasing blood flow.[31]

There are many other mechanisms by which PRP may aid hair growth. Li et al showed increased levels of β-catenin, extracellular signal-related kinase, and Akt signaling, all of which contribute to dermal papilla cell proliferation.[12] Activated PRP increased levels of phosphorylated extracellular signal regulated kinases and phosphorylated Akt, molecules which resulted in human dermal papilla propagation.[12] Interestingly, the effects of PRP were found to be dose dependent in this study, indicating the importance of attaining appropriate levels of PRP to achieve maximum results.

Numerous studies have detailed PRP and its anti-apoptotic effects.[32,33] This mechanism is based on the ability of PRP to induce activation of Bcl-2 and phosphorylation of Akt, both involved in antiapoptotic regulation. Dermal papilla cells are protected from premature breakdown and remain active, thereby extending the anagen phase of the hair cycle and delaying induction into catagen and telogen phases.[34,35,36] Further-more, Li et al found that PRP treatment almost doubled β- catenin transcriptional activity, which is expressed in the anagen hair follicle. This, along with PRP's ability to upregulate fibroblast growth factor 7 (FGF-7), also aids in lengthening the anagen or growth phase of the hair cycle, as well.[12,32] Finally, promoting FGF-7 signaling has also been shown to promote stem cell differentiation into hair follicles.[37]

1.4 Mechanism of Action for PRP on Rejuvenation and Repair

Like hair growth, there are likely several mechanisms by which PRP influences skin rejuvenation. Accumulated fragmented collagen fibrils prevent new collagen growth and lead to extracellular matrix breakdown.[38] Activated PRP increases expression of matrix metallopeptidase (MMP-1 and MMP-3), stimulating extracellular membrane remodeling and removal of damaged collagen fragments, ultimately allowing for improved, more regularly organized collagen synthesis.[39,40] PRP contains multiple growth factors that stimulate human dermal fibroblasts and boost neocollagenesis.[40] It has also been shown to enhance the secretion of hyaluronic acid.[41] Among its many functions in the dermis, hyaluronic acid avidly binds water, thereby increasing skin volume and hydration. Taken together, these findings suggest that the PRP solution may augment extracellular matrix synthesis and is a possible treatment for skin rejuvenation and acne scaring.[42]

PRP has recently been used with resurfacing ablative lasers to treat facial acne scaring. It has also been used for wound care post ablative laser treatments.[23] Ablative carbon dioxide fractional laser resurfacing has been shown to produce

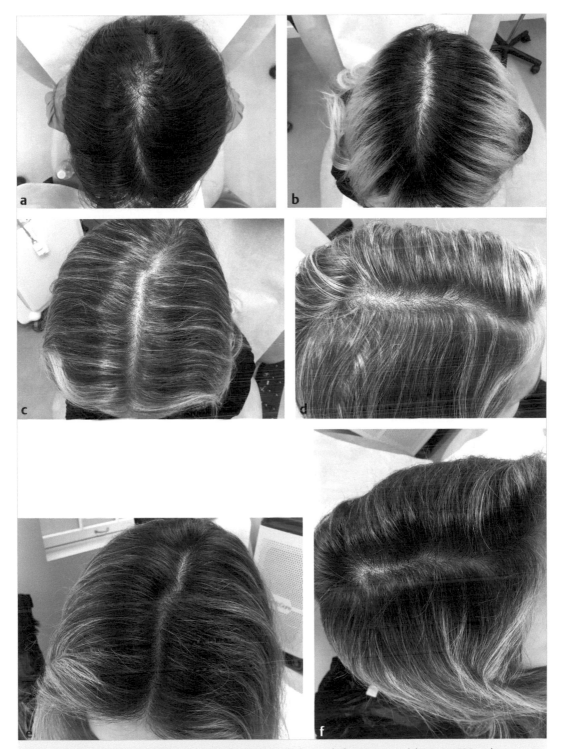

Fig. 1.1 Platelet-rich plasma (PRP) used in female hair loss—before and after. Patient 1 **(a)** prior to PRP and **(b)** 4 months post treatment. Patient 2 **(c, d)** prior to PRP and **(e, f)** 4 months post treatment.

similar pathology to that of normal wounds. As such, adding platelets, a key element to normal wound repair, should assist and hasten tissue regeneration after ablative laser therapy.[43] While unproven at this time, it is believed that PRP's release of α-granules containing large storage pools of growth factors, leads to more efficient and expedited tissue healing. Additionally, PRP was shown to expedite wound healing, reduce erythema, and decrease transepidermal water loss in patients post fractional ablative resurfacing.

1.5 Options for Preparation

Abstraction of PRP relies on differential centrifugation of whole blood and separation of the desired components based on their specific gravity. PRP preparation can be done either manually or by automated device. Regardless, the basic process begins by drawing peripheral blood from the patient (▶ Fig. 1.2a–e). The tubes of blood (often containing an anticoagulant agent) are then spun in a centrifuge, according to proprietary protocols with set speed, spin cycles, and spin times. Rapid spinning layers the different blood cell lines based on mass so that platelets in plasma—hence the name platelet-rich plasma (PRP)—can be extracted from the tubes with variable concentrations of erythrocytes and granulocytes (▶ Fig. 1.3). Some protocols add activating substances (see below) prior to use.[44]

The two main methods of manual PRP preparation are the "PRP production" method and the "buffy coat" method. In the "PRP production" method, whole blood undergoes an initial slower centrifugation, called a "soft spin," which yields an upper layer consisting of platelets and leukocytes, a middle layer, called a buffy coat (which is rich in white blood cells [WBCs]) and a bottom layer, containing mostly red blood cells (RBC). The upper layer and superficial buffy coat are then extracted and undergo a second round of centrifugation at a higher speed, called a "hard spin". This results in the formation of soft pellets mainly composed of platelets, along with platelet-poor plasma (PPP), which is then removed, leaving PRP.[45]

In the "buffy coat" method, whole blood is first undergoes a heavy spin, separating it into a top layer of PPP, a buffy coat middle layer (containing PRP), and RBC on the bottom. Supernatant plasma is removed and the buffy coat is then given a soft spin, yielding pure PRP and leukocytes, which are disposed.[44]

Currently, there are several automated, commercial PRP production systems available that facilitate PRP production in an efficient and simple process. Automated systems use sensors to distinguish the buffy coat–RBC interface. This results in a consistent concentration of PRP produced. Each system uses a different method to collect and concentrate platelets. Generally, 30 mL of whole blood will yield 3 to 5 mL of PRP (depending on the patient's platelet level, system and technique used).[44] Automated production of PRP is not consistent in its results, but has greater reproducibility than manual methods. Additionally, closed systems reduce possible errors and help ensure sterile conditions are maintained throughout the entirety of the procedure.[46]

Before injection, PRP is often activated by the addition of thrombin or calcium chloride. Once activated, PRP must be used immediately to maintain its viability.[3] Some systems do not require this step since collagen is a natural activator of PRP and, therefore, does not require exogenous activation when used in soft tissue.[44]

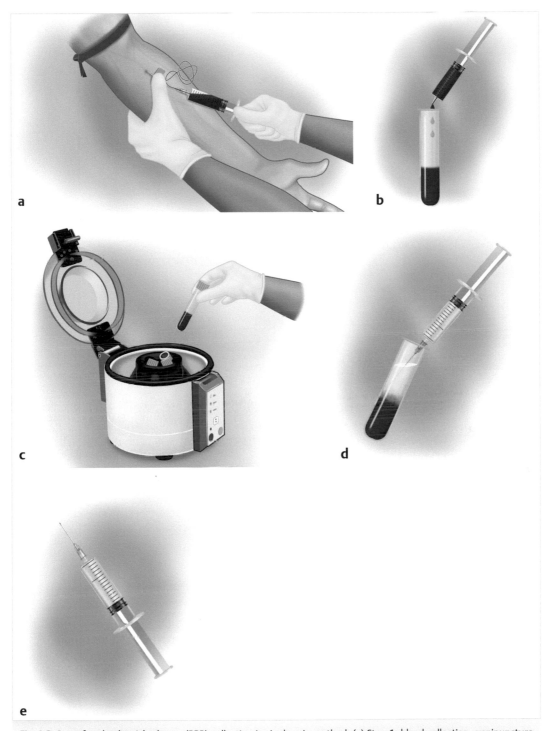

Fig. 1.2 Steps for platelet-rich plasma (PRP) collection in single spin method. (a) Step 1: blood collection—venipuncture from antecubital vein. (b) Step 2: transfer blood into collection tubes for centrifugation. (c) Step 3: place specimens in centrifuge. (d) Step 4: withdrawing PRP layer into syringe post centrifugation. (e) Step 5: syringe with PRP only ready for injection.

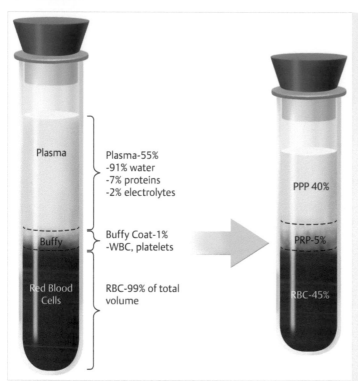

Plasma

Plasma-55%
-91% water
-7% proteins
-2% electrolytes

PPP 40%

Buffy

Buffy Coat-1%
-WBC, platelets

PRP-5%

Red Blood
Cells

RBC-99% of total
volume

RBC-45%

Fig. 1.3 Makeup of whole blood and platelet-rich plasma.

1.5.1 Practical Considerations when Evaluating PRP Systems

When selecting a PRP preparation system appraisal, there are many variables to consider. Each proprietary system currently available varies widely regarding their method of preparation. There is no guideline or standard as to the appropriate technique to achieve the optimal platelet concentration in PRP preparations.[32] This makes comparing and evaluating systems difficult. However, certain criteria must be considered when determining which to use in a given practice setting.[47]

It is critical to take note of the platelet concentrations produced by each system. While the optimal concentration for dermatologic or plastic surgery indications is still unknown, different systems produce highly variable solutions.[44] As noted previously, it has been shown that at minimal, 1,000,000 platelets/µl are needed for wound healing and 1,500,000 platelets/µl are optimal for angiogenesis (▶ Table 1.3).[13,15]

There is much debate regarding the impact of WBCs in PRP. Many believe that WBC are important components of PRP due to their antimicrobial properties that protect against infections and potential allergies.[48] Others maintain that platelets already contain anti-microbial properties and therefore WBC are unnecessary. In fact, it has also been suggested the presence of elevated levels of WBCs, specifically neutrophils, may be detrimental to the healing process. Neutrophils cause inflammation, potentially damaging non-injured tissue, resulting in undesired fibrosis, scaring, and catabolic cascades.[49,50] Additionally, concentrated leukocytes can counteract many of the growth factors released in close proximity.[51] These effects have been shown to hinder wound healing.[48] As such, Sundman et al note that in addition to the concentration of

Table 1.3 Comparison of preparation systems

System	Mean platelet concentration ($\times 10^9$/L)	Mean WBC ($\times 10^9$/L)	Mean neutrophils ($\times 10^9$/L)	Mean RBC ($\times 10^9$/L)
Control	269	8.73	5.5	4.7
Magellan (Arteriocyte Medical)	1266	31.4	15.1	1.03
GPS III (Biomet)	964	35.8	15.4	1.03
ACP (Athrex)	412	1.3	0.4	0.0333
SmartPrep2 (Harvest)	1224	24.7	6.47	1.43

Source: Adapted from Fitzpatrick, J, Bulsara, MK, McCrory, PR, Richardson, MD, Zheng, MH. Analysis of platelet-rich plasma extraction variations in platelet and blood components between 4 common commercial kits. Orthop J Sports Med. 2017;5(1):2325967116675272.

platelets, the efficacy of PRP is also dependent on obtaining the appropriate ratio of platelets to WBC. Plasma-based method employs a shorter, slower spin with the goal of removing WBC, in exchange for losing some platelets. The buffy coat method uses a longer spin with a higher rate to create a buffy coat and capture as many platelets as possible.[52] Red blood contain reactive oxygen species, which produce unwanted inflammatory reactions where injected. RBCs injected directly into tissue would likely result in increased edema and pain for the patient.[50] Furthermore, inflammation has a negative impact on hair regrowth. It creates a catabolic environment that does not promote regeneration and hinders the effects of growth factors. It may be also induce telogen effluvium, an unwanted outcome. Multiple studies have shown that each system produces varying quantities of WBCs and RBCs, despite similar preparation techniques (▶ Table 1.3).[53,54] As such, further studies comparing the various systems are necessary.

When comparing systems, it is important to note that different devices use different volumes, making concentration measurements unreliable. As such, preparation systems should always be evaluated using total dose of platelets. Additionally, it is vital to find a system that produces undamaged platelets, since platelet disruption yields diminished growth factor production.[13] Spin time, centrifugal acceleration, and distance between the proteins are all key factors contributing the quality and thus, efficacy of prepare PRP. Additional factors worth considering include the centrifuge rotor (ease and smoothness of spin), anticoagulant used or means for preventing platelet aggregation (for instance, acidity can influence both comfort when injected and platelet quality), and minimization of the platelet gradient. Efficient conditions for platelet recovery are low centrifugal acceleration (close to $100 \times g$, 10 minutes) in the first spin and around $400 \times g$ in the second spin for preventing effects on activating platelets.[48]

There is much conflicting data about the efficacy of single vs dual spin PRP preparations. In theory, single spin (plasma methods) should produce lower concentrations of platelets that double spin (buffy coat) methods. While there are studies that support this,[55] there are other studies that have shown single spin systems to be effective in concentrating platelets in PRP to adequate levels.[53] It should also be noted that both studies had high standard deviations, indicating high levels of variability. There are multiple systems available that employ differing spin methods. For example, the Eclipse and RegenLabs use a single spin method (▶ Fig. 1.2a–e). Additionally, new systems on the market now claim to be able to accomplish dual spinning within one centrifuge appliance (▶ Fig. 1.4a–e). Each individual system

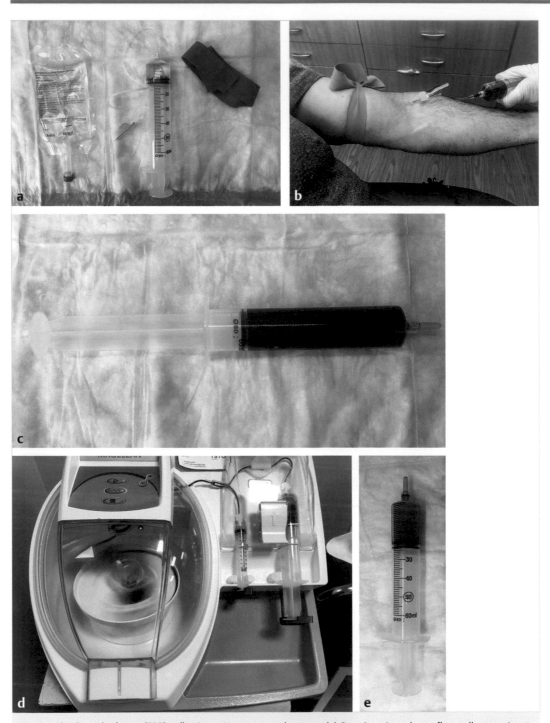

Fig. 1.4 Platelet-rich plasma (PRP) collection using automated system. **(a)** Step 1: syringe, butterfly needle, tourniquet, and anticoagulant for phlebotomy. **(b)** Step 2: drawing blood from antecubital vein. **(c)** Step 3: blood mixed with anticoagulant ready for centrifugation. **(d)** Step 4: centrifugation of blood. **(e)** Step 5: PRP ready for injection.

must be evaluated independently to determine the true level of platelet concentration. There are multiple additional factors that come into play. The use of some anesthetics and anticoagulants may alter the pH, creating a suboptimal pH for PRP. There is a study that also shows varying effects based on the metals used in the centrifuge.[52] Further independent studies are needed to formally investigate each individual criteria in each of the PRP systems available on the market.

The utilization of PRP in an aesthetic setting has unique requirements when compared to other specialties. The quantity of PRP produced is dependent on the volume of blood drawn and the capacity of the centrifuge per spin. Orthopedic and other surgical systems require spinning large quantities of blood to produce the quantity needed for extensive surgeries. This technique may be appropriate for use during reconstructive or plastic surgery procedures in the operating room. However, point-of-care, in-office dermatologic applications generally require approximately 5 to 12 mL of PRP, so finding a system that spins the appropriate, smaller volume of blood is necessary. Small vials, however, have a limited concentrating capacity, since only a fraction of the drawn blood becomes PRP and in general, the more concentrated the solution, the lower the overall yield. Size of the centrifuge, cost of consumables, and time required for collection and processing require consideration as well. Outpatient practices prefer compact centrifuge systems, in contrast to hospital operating room systems that have fewer space constraints. Consumable costs must be considered due to the multiple treatment protocols for many dermatologic conditions. As such, maintaining a reasonable price point for patients is important to ensure feasibility and sustain long-term compliance with treatment protocols. Shorter spin times are also favorable in this fast pace, office setting.

Manual systems are enticing to the practitioner because they are inexpensive and purport to achieve high PRP concentrations. However, these systems are highly technique dependent, have the potential for contamination, are susceptible to platelet damage, and require more hands on time to fully prepare. Automated systems, although more expensive, streamline the preparation process, minimize damage to platelets, and decrease the possibility of contamination.[46]

1.6 Conclusion

The use of PRP in aesthetic dermatologic and plastic surgery practices has surged. PRP is an autologous solution containing concentrated platelets that on activation sets off a cascade of growth factors and triggers neovascularization, tissue remodeling, and anti-apoptosis pathways. It is crucial to understand the advantages and disadvantages of different preparation systems and identify which methods produce the highest yield, best quality PRP. Future randomized clinical studies will delineate the role of PRP in many cosmetic applications. It is likely that the ideal system will differ based on clinical condition.

References

[1] Pierce GF, Mustoe TA, Lingelbach J, et al. Platelet-derived growth factor and transforming growth factor-beta enhance tissue repair activities by unique mechanisms. J Cell Biol. 1989; 109(1):429–440

[2] Oz MC, Jeevanandam V, Smith CR, et al. Autologous fibrin glue from intraoperatively collected platelet-rich plasma. Ann Thorac Surg. 1992; 53(3):530–531

[3] Mishra A, Woodall J, Jr, Vieira A. Treatment of tendon and muscle using platelet-rich plasma. Clin Sports Med. 2009; 28 (1):113–125

[4] Kang JS, Zheng Z, Choi MJ, Lee SH, Kim DY, Cho SB. The effect of CD34 + cell-containing autologous platelet-rich plasma injection on pattern hair loss: a preliminary study. J Eur Acad Dermatol Venereol. 2014; 28(1):72–79

[5] Adler SC, Kent KJ. Enhancing wound healing with growth factors. Facial Plast Surg Clin North Am. 2002; 10(2):129–146

[6] Leo MS, Kumar AS, Kirit R, Konathan R, Sivamani RK. Systematic review of the use of platelet-rich plasma in aesthetic dermatology. J Cosmet Dermatol. 2015; 14(4):315–323

[7] Lynch MD, Bashir S. Applications of platelet-rich plasma in dermatology: A critical appraisal of the literature. J Dermatolog Treat. 2016; 27(3):285–289

[8] Arshdeep, Kumaran MS. Platelet-rich plasma in dermatology: boon or a bane? Indian J Dermatol Venereol Leprol. 2014; 80 (1):5–14

[9] Kon E, Filardo G, Di Martino A, Marcacci M. Platelet-rich plasma (PRP) to treat sports injuries: evidence to support its use. Knee Surg Sports Traumatol Arthrosc. 2011; 19(4):516–527

[10] Andia I, Maffulli N. Platelet-rich plasma for managing pain and inflammation in osteoarthritis. Nat Rev Rheumatol. 2013; 9(12):721–730

[11] Tözüm TF, Demiralp B. Platelet-rich plasma: a promising innovation in dentistry. J Can Dent Assoc. 2003; 69(10): 664–664

[12] Li ZJ, Choi HI, Choi DK, et al. Autologous platelet-rich plasma: a potential therapeutic tool for promoting hair growth. Dermatol Surg. 2012; 38(7 Pt 1):1040–1046

[13] Marx RE. Platelet-rich plasma (PRP): what is PRP and what is not PRP? Implant Dent. 2001; 10(4):225–228

[14] Eppley BL, Woodell JE, Higgins J. Platelet quantification and growth factor analysis from platelet-rich plasma: implications for wound healing. Plast Reconstr Surg. 2004; 114(6): 1502–1508

[15] Giusti I, Rughetti A, D'Ascenzo S, et al. Identification of an optimal concentration of platelet gel for promoting angiogenesis in human endothelial cells. Transfusion. 2009; 49(4):771–778

[16] Weibrich G, Hansen T, Kleis W, Buch R, Hitzler WE. Effect of platelet concentration in platelet-rich plasma on peri-implant bone regeneration. Bone. 2004; 34(4):665–671

[17] Sánchez AR, Sheridan PJ, Kupp LI. Is platelet-rich plasma the perfect enhancement factor? A current review. Int J Oral Maxillofac Implants. 2003; 18(1):93–103

[18] Marx RE. Platelet-rich plasma: evidence to support its use. J Oral Maxillofac Surg. 2004; 62(4):489–496

[19] Eppley BL, Pietrzak WS, Blanton M. Platelet-rich plasma: a review of biology and applications in plastic surgery. Plast Reconstr Surg. 2006; 118(6):147e–159e

[20] Takikawa M, Nakamura S, Nakamura S, et al. Enhanced effect of platelet-rich plasma containing a new carrier on hair growth. Dermatol Surg. 2011; 37(12):1721–1729

[21] Khatu SS, More YE, Gokhale NR, Chavhan DC, Bendsure N. Platelet-rich plasma in androgenic alopecia: myth or an effective tool. J Cutan Aesthet Surg. 2014; 7(2):107–110

[22] Crovetti G, Martinelli G, Issi M, et al. Platelet gel for healing cutaneous chronic wounds. Transfus Apheresis Sci. 2004; 30 (2):145–151

[23] Na JI, Choi JW, Choi HR, et al. Rapid healing and reduced erythema after ablative fractional carbon dioxide laser resurfacing combined with the application of autologous platelet-rich plasma. Dermatol Surg. 2011; 37(4):463–468

[24] Steed DL. The role of growth factors in wound healing. Surg Clin North Am. 1997; 77(3):575–586

[25] Sunitha Raja V, Munirathnam Naidu E. Platelet-rich fibrin: evolution of a second-generation platelet concentrate. Indian J Dent Res. 2008; 19(1):42–46

[26] Lee KS, Wilson JJ, Rabago DP, Baer GS, Jacobson JA, Borrero CG. Musculoskeletal applications of platelet-rich plasma: fad or future? AJR Am J Roentgenol. 2011; 196(3):628–636

[27] Mecklenburg L, Tobin DJ, Müller-Röver S, et al. Active hair growth (anagen) is associated with angiogenesis. J Invest Dermatol. 2000; 114(5):909–916

[28] Tarallo V, Vesci L, Capasso O, et al. A placental growth factor variant unable to recognize vascular endothelial growth factor (VEGF) receptor-1 inhibits VEGF-dependent tumor angiogenesis via heterodimerization. Cancer Res. 2010; 70(5): 1804–1813

[29] Cervelli V, Garcovich S, Bielli A, et al. The effect of autologous activated platelet rich plasma (AA-PRP) injection on pattern hair loss: clinical and histomorphometric evaluation. BioMed Res Int. 2014; 2014:760709

[30] Uebel CO, da Silva JB, Cantarelli D, Martins P. The role of platelet plasma growth factors in male pattern baldness surgery. Plast Reconstr Surg. 2006; 118(6):1458–1466, discussion 1467

[31] Li W, Enomoto M, Ukegawa M, et al. Subcutaneous injections of platelet-rich plasma into skin flaps modulate proangiogenic gene expression and improve survival rates. Plast Reconstr Surg. 2012; 129(4):858–866

[32] Maria-Angeliki G, Alexandros-Efstratios K, Dimitris R, Konstantinos K. Platelet-rich plasma as a potential treatment for noncicatricial alopecias. Int J Trichology. 2015; 7(2):54–63

[33] Kwon OS, Pyo HK, Oh YJ, et al. Promotive effect of minoxidil combined with all-trans retinoic acid (tretinoin) on human hair growth in vitro. J Korean Med Sci. 2007; 22(2): 283–289

[34] Ferraris C, Cooklis M, Polakowska RR, Haake AR. Induction of apoptosis through the PKC pathway in cultured dermal papilla fibroblasts. Exp Cell Res. 1997; 234(1):37–46

[35] Park KY, Kim IS, Kim BJ, Kim MN. Letter: autologous fat grafting and platelet-rich plasma for treatment of facial contour defects. Dermatol Surg. 2012; 38(9):1572–1574

[36] Krasna M, Domanović D, Tomsic A, Svajger U, Jeras M. Platelet gel stimulates proliferation of human dermal fibroblasts in vitro. Acta Dermatovenerol Alp Panonica Adriat. 2007; 16(3): 105–110

[37] Sohn KC, Shi G, Jang S, et al. Pitx2, a beta-catenin-regulated transcription factor, regulates the differentiation of outer root sheath cells cultured in vitro. J Dermatol Sci. 2009; 54(1): 6–11

[38] Jenkins G. Molecular mechanisms of skin ageing. Mech Ageing Dev. 2002; 123(7):801–810

[39] Kim DH, Je YJ, Kim CD, et al. Can platelet-rich plasma be used for skin rejuvenation? Evaluation of effects of platelet-rich plasma on human dermal fibroblast. Ann Dermatol. 2011; 23 (4):424–431

[40] Cho JW, Kim SA, Lee KS. Platelet-rich plasma induces increased expression of G1 cell cycle regulators, type I collagen, and matrix metalloproteinase-1 in human skin fibroblasts. Int J Mol Med. 2012; 29(1):32–36

[41] Anitua E, Sánchez M, Nurden AT, et al. Platelet-released growth factors enhance the secretion of hyaluronic acid and induce hepatocyte growth factor production by synovial fibroblasts from arthritic patients. Rheumatology (Oxford). 2007; 46(12):1769–1772

[42] Gawdat HI, Hegazy RA, Fawzy MM, Fathy M. Autologous platelet rich plasma: topical versus intradermal after fractional ablative carbon dioxide laser treatment of atrophic acne scars. Dermatol Surg. 2014; 40(2):152–161

[43] Lee JW, Kim BJ, Kim MN, Mun SK. The efficacy of autologous platelet rich plasma combined with ablative carbon dioxide fractional resurfacing for acne scars: a simultaneous split-face trial. Dermatol Surg. 2011; 37(7):931–938

[44] Dhurat R, Sukesh M. Principles and Methods of Preparation of Platelet-Rich Plasma: A Review and Author's Perspective. J Cutan Aesthet Surg. 2014; 7(4):189–197

[45] Sweeny J, Grossman BJ. Blood collection, storage and component preparation methods. In: Brecher M, ed. Technical Manual. 14th ed. Bethesda, MD: American Association of Blood Banks (AABB); 2002:955–8

[46] Fontenot RL, Sink CA, Werre SR, Weinstein NM, Dahlgren LA. Simple tube centrifugation for processing platelet-rich plasma in the horse. Can Vet J. 2012; 53(12):1266–1272

[47] Mehta V. Platelet-rich plasma: a review of the science and possible clinical applications. Orthopedics. 2010; 33(2):111

[48] Perez AGM, Lana JFSD, Rodrigues AA, Luzo ACM, Belangero WD, Santana MHA. Relevant aspects of centrifugation step in the preparation of platelet-rich plasma. ISRN Hematol. 2014; 2014:176060

[49] Fitzpatrick J, Bulsara MK, McCrory PR, Richardson MD, Zheng MH. Analysis of platelet-rich plasma extraction variations in platelet and blood components between 4 common commercial kits. Orthop J Sports Med. 2017; 5(1):2325967116675272

[50] Magalon J, Bausset O, Serratrice N, et al. Characterization and comparison of 5 platelet-rich plasma preparations in a single-donor model. Arthroscopy. 2014; 30(5):629–638

[51] Sundman EA, Cole BJ, Fortier LA. Growth factor and catabolic cytokine concentrations are influenced by the cellular composition of platelet-rich plasma. Am J Sports Med. 2011; 39 (10):2135–2140

[52] DeLong JM, Russell RP, Mazzocca AD. Platelet-rich plasma: the PAW classification system. Arthroscopy. 2012; 28(7):998–1009

[53] Mazzocca AD, McCarthy MB, Chowaniec DM, et al. Platelet-rich plasma differs according to preparation method and human variability. J Bone Joint Surg Am. 2012; 94(4):308–316

[54] Castillo TN, Pouliot MA, Kim HJ, Dragoo JL. Comparison of growth factor and platelet concentration from commercial platelet-rich plasma separation systems. Am J Sports Med. 2011; 39(2):266–271

[55] Nagata MJ, Messora MR, Furlaneto FA, et al. Effectiveness of two methods for preparation of autologous platelet-rich plasma: an experimental study in rabbits. Eur J Dent. 2010; 4(4): 395–402

2

Platelet-Rich Plasma and Fibrin Sealants in Plastic Surgery: Clinical Applications and One Practice's Experience

Kamakshi Zeidler and R. Lawrence Berkowitz

Abstract

Platelet products have been used intraoperatively both as a solution (platelet-rich plasma [PRP]) and as an autologous sealant (platelet-rich fibrin matrix). Sealants may be particularly useful in aesthetic facial surgeries, as demonstrated in our practice and a growing, albeit small, body of literature showing lower rates of hematoma and/or seroma as well as more rapid return to socialization than anticipated. The data surrounding addition of PRP to autologous fat grafting is mixed. Inconsistent findings may result from differences in PRP purity and preparation methodology, resulting in variable solutions that may positively or negatively impact delicate grafts depending on the composition. Further large-scale, randomized, controlled studies are necessary to confirm these preliminary, especially since such aesthetic procedures are elective, so any therapies that optimize outcomes and speed recovery are welcome.

Keywords: platelet-rich plasma, platelet-poor plasma, platelet-rich fibrin matrix/platelet-rich fibrin sealant, plastic surgery, aesthetic facial surgery, rhinoplasty, facelift, endoscopic brow lift, blepharoplasty, otoplasty, laser resurfacing, fat grafting, hematoma, seroma

Key Points

- Platelet products have been used intraoperatively both as a solution (platelet-rich plasma [PRP]) and as an autologous sealant (platelet-rich fibrin matrix).
- We have had excellent outcomes using platelet-poor fibrin sealant then PRP during all open or endoscopic facial surgery including rhinoplasty with or without septoplasty, face and neck lift, minimal access cranial suspension short scar facelift, endoscopic brow lift, blepharoplasty, otoplasty, and laser resurfacing.
- Our rates of hematoma and/or seroma as well as recovery time (return to socialization) are substantially less than anticipated. A growing body of literature supports these findings, though many studies have been underpowered.
- In terms of autologous fat grafting, addition of PRP has yielded variable results, perhaps due to differences in PRP purity and preparation methodology.

Since learning of the availability of platelet-rich plasma (PRP) as an autologous fibrin sealant (platelet-rich fibrin sealant or platelet-rich fibrin matrix) in 2001,[1] the senior author has used multiple PRP preparation systems. The concept of an autologous product that would both act as a sealant as well as promote wound healing was intriguing. Prior to 2001, this technology was known to oral and maxillofacial surgeons, otolaryngologists, and orthopedists but just being introduced into the plastic surgery literature.[2,3] The role of platelets in wound healing had been recognized for decades, but before the early 2000s, we were only familiar with using platelet concentrates to accelerate reepithelialization (where delay in wound healing had occurred in cases of lathyrism from the effects of medications used to treat rheumatoid arthritis).[4]

In our practice, this product has been useful as a sealant for open surgical procedures and to accelerate the wound healing process. It is uncommonly used for body procedures such as mammoplasty and abdominoplasty since the volume required for such large surface areas makes it impractical. However, platelet products lend themselves quite well to facial procedures because of the smaller surface area, specifically rhinoplasty, facelifts, endoscopic brow lifts, blepharoplasty, otoplasty, and laser resurfacing.[5,6,7] These operations rely on perfect hemostasis for ideal aesthetic outcomes and therefore, it is critical to avoid the sequelae of postoperative bleeding. Even small collections of blood can result in fibrosis and deformities. In our practice, the routine utilization of PRP as an autologous fibrin sealant has fulfilled this promise by helping to reduce bleeding and speed recovery. Patients benefit from the reliable hemostasis and jumpstart in the healing process; in particular, facelift patients do not need surgical drains, and many enjoy a rapid return to society including work, school, and social life. This reduced recovery time makes facial rejuvenation and nasal reshaping procedures more palatable to our patients. Downtime for surgical recovery due to ecchymosis and swelling has always been a barrier to patients seeking these otherwise life-changing procedures. We have a long experience with the use of other medications and surgical instruments whose function is to reduce ecchymosis and swelling including desmopressin (DDAVP) as a hemostatic agent and ultrahigh-frequency power tools (Piezotome; Comeg Medical, Minneapolis, MN) for precision reshaping of bone and cartilage.[8,9,10] Minimizing recovery while optimizing outcomes may have a profound impact. So, all adjuncts to surgery such as PRP, that decrease downtime should be implemented.

We share our vast experience using platelet products intraoperatively followed by discussion of the evidence to date.

2.1 Methods and Materials

All patients undergoing an open or endoscopic facial surgery including rhinoplasty with or without septoplasty, endoscopic brow lift, face and neck lift, minimal access cranial suspension short scar facelift, blepharoplasty, otoplasty, and laser resurfacing were treated with platelet-poor fibrin sealant and then PRP following the manufacturer's guidelines. The patients were screened for anticoagulant medications and supplements and discontinued from these starting two weeks prior to surgery. They were instructed to abstain from alcohol for 24 hours prior to the procedure. Untreated or undertreated hypertension was addressed by primary care physician prior to the operation. All patients on angiotensin-converting enzyme inhibitors or angiotensin II receptor blockers were switched to a β-blocker perioperatively to avoid angioedema. All patients underwent an autologous blood draw following strict Harvest protocol and strict sterile technique. Blood draw was usually at the time of intravenous catheter insertion utilizing a 20-gauge catheter. This was done before any intravenous medications were administered. When catheter extraction of the required aliquot became difficult due to vein collapse, then the blood was drawn in the operating room after the induction of general anesthesia when veins generally dilate. The collected volume depended on the need for a small Harvest kit (AdiPrep II system, Harvest Terumo BCT, Inc., Lakewood, CO) for rhinoplasty, blepharoplasty, otoplasty or periorbital laser resurfacing or large kit for facelift, endoscopic brow lift, or full-face laser resurfacing, based on necessary body surface area. The blood draw was done with the requisite 30-cc or 60-cc syringe, respectively and mixed with a citrate anticoagulant to prevent clot formation. Preparation followed the manufacturer instructions. Briefly, blood was transferred to a sterile double barrel receptacle for underwent two centrifuge spin cycles—the first for 11 minutes and second for 3 minutes. We extracted platelet-poor plasma (PPP) from the top layer of the centrifuge specimen and injected into a sterile cup on the sterile operating field. A small Harvest generally yields 10 cc of PPP and the larger Harvest 20 cc of PPP. Next, the bottom of PRP portion was extracted and injected into a separate sterile cup on the field. With a small Harvest, we expect approximately 3 cc of PRP and a large, 6 cc of PRP. Topical thrombin (of bovine origin) was placed in a third cup on the sterile field and mixed with calcium gluconate provided the necessary catalyst to initiate the fibrin cascade. The two products are delivered via a double

barrel syringe (a 10 mL for the plasma either PPP or PRP, and a 1 mL for the thrombin calcium solution). The spray emitted through the double-barrel syringes was delivered via one of two applicator tip options: one with two small openings (for wide field use such as facelifts and laser resurfacing) and the other with a catheter tip (for narrow surgical fields such as endoscopic procedures, rhinoplasty, or septoplasty use). A fibrin clot forms, when the substances contact the open wound. In all cases, a fine mist was sprayed over the entire field with PPP fibrin sealant then followed by gentle compression of the tissues over the wound bed for 5 minutes. We expected a sealant not an adhesive effect, observing a tacky consistency. Finally, a fine mist of the PRP fibrin sealant was sprayed over the wound bed, paying attention to good coverage of the incision sites, to promote wound healing.

Of note, we have since switched preparatory systems and in fact, have multiple in our office. The number of FDA-cleared class II devices has increased in number since implementation of our off-label protocol. We have achieved good results using various protocols, although have not compared them head-to-head. Discussion of preparatory protocols and systems is beyond the scope of this section and addressed more fully in Chapter 1.

The 58 consecutive face and neck lift patients including the short scar and full incisional techniques, and 64 consecutive rhinoplasties with or without septoplasty that were completed between January 2017 and June 2018 were included in the analysis. We did not include endoscopic brow lift or resurfacing procedures in this analysis (see Chapter 3 for laser resurfacing). There were no exclusion criteria other than the suitability of the patient to undergo such facial procedures. The gender distribution for facelift was 3 male and 55 female, and for rhinoplasty, 15 male and 49 female. The majority of rhinoplasties included septoplasty and turbinate reduction with radiofrequency devices. In the cases of face and neck lift (▶ Table 2.1 and ▶ Table 2.2), hematoma, infection, skin compromise, ecchymosis, and time considered adequate for social reintegration were taken from the patient's record. In the cases of rhinoplasty (▶ Table 2.3 and ▶ Table 2.4), hematoma (septal or subcutaneous), ecchymosis, and suitability for return to socialization are recorded as extracted from the patient's record.

Table 2.1 Complications and wound healing after facelift

Postoperative condition	Incidence (*n*, total 58)	Percentage (%)
Hematoma[a]	0	0.0
Microhematoma[b]	1	1.7
Infection	1	1.7
Skin compromise	1	1.7
Ecchymoses	50	86.2
No or minimal ecchymoses[c]	8	13.8

[a]Requiring surgical intervention.
[b]Aspirated with needle and syringe in office.
[c]Always associated with cases of facelift only without autologous fat grafting.

Table 2.2 Return to full socialization after facelift[a]

Duration (weeks)	Incidence (*n*, total 58)	Percentage (%)
1	1	1.7
2	22	37.9
3	34	58.6
4	1	1.1

[a]Defined as return to social gatherings, work, or school. No patient required more than 4 weeks to achieve these criteria.

Table 2.3 Complications and wound healing after rhinoplasty

Postoperative condition	Incidence (*n*, total 64)	Percentage (%)
Hematoma[a]	0	0.0
Epistaxis[b]	0	0.0
Ecchymoses[c]	24	37.5

[a]Defined as either septal or subcutaneous.
[b]Defined as requiring surgical intervention to control.
[c]Defined as such that either intense pulse light or laser treatment required and/or camouflage to cover.

Table 2.4 Return to full socialization after rhinoplasty[a]

Duration (weeks)	Incidence (n, total 58)	Percentage (%)
1	42	64.0
2	23	36.0

[a]Defined as return to social activities, school, or work. No patient required more than 2 weeks.

2.2 Results

For facelift (full- or short-scar techniques) procedures, we observed no cases of hematoma or seroma. No drains were employed in any of these cases. Ecchymosis was still present to some degree in most, especially when autologous fat grafting was used as an adjunct (which was performed in the majority of patients). In cases without autologous fat grafting where the blunt trauma from a cannula was minimal, occasionally, there were no ecchymoses, as reflected in ▶ Table 2.1. Tissue compromise behind the ears was rare in full face and neck lift with one significant delay of healing in a patient determined to have Raynaud's disease postoperatively. Return to socialization was gradual with the use of camouflage makeup and intense pulse light (BBL; Sciton Inc., Mountain View, CA) at 515 nm or pulse-dye laser (V-Beam Perfecta; Syneron Candela, Wayland, MA) treatments to aid in the rapid recovery and resolution of ecchymoses. All patients were able to return to work, school, or social activities by the end of 3 weeks. A few, especially those who did not undergo fat grafting, were cleared of obvious stigmata by 2 weeks, and rarely, a highly motivated patient would reenter society at 1 week (► Table 2.2). These findings are in contradistinction to the widely reported and expected 1% to 3% incidents of hematoma in females and up to 7 to 9% in males.[11,12,13]

For rhinoplasty, which has a reputation for prolonged recovery lasting up to 6 weeks or longer, the results have been remarkable (► Table 2.3 and ► Table 2.4). It must be stressed, however, that all rhinoplasty patients also received desmopressin (DDAVP) to reduce bleeding and that ultrahigh-frequency power tools (Stryker Corporation; Kalamazoo, MI or more recently, Piezo ultrasonic devices) were always employed in place of rasps and hammer-driven osteotomes. These power tools are more precise and known to reduce trauma and ecchymosis in rhinoplasty surgery. The vast majority of procedures were done as open rhinoplasty, allowing for full field visualization and hemostasis with bipolar cautery. The risk of hematoma has been reported in rhinoplasty as 0.2% and epistaxis approximately 2%. In contrast, we had no reported cases of either during the follow-up period.

2.3 Discussion of Platelet-Rich Plasma and Fibrin in Facial Surgery

The use of fibrin sealants and PRP has proven useful in a variety of head and neck plastic surgery procedures. We report substantially lower than anticipated rates of hematoma and/or seroma.

For example, in facelift surgery, the rate of hematoma is generally estimated to be 1 to 3% in females and as high as 7 to 9% in males.[11,12,13] The elimination of drains frequently employed in facelift procedures makes the process more tolerable for patients and caregivers with a faster return to normal activity—no longer than 3 weeks. In the cases of rhinoplasty, with or without septoplasty, our patients had fewer ecchymoses, especially when coupled with other useful adjuncts. Most patients are partially socialized at the end of 1 week and fully socialized at 2 weeks, a substantially accelerated recovery timeline. Of note, for rhinoplasty, the use of fibrin sealants and PRP is always used in conjunction with other adjunct therapies, so it is impossible to estimate the relative contribution of each on recovery. While there is a paucity of data and those that exist are largely underpowered studies, a 2017 meta-analysis of 2,434 patients undergoing facelift procedures is the best peer reviewed data available and corroborates our small, uncontrolled study. It showed a statistically significant reduction in the incidence of hematoma (risk ratio, 0.37; 95% confidence interval, 0.18–0.74; $p = 0.005$) and wound drainage ($p < 0.001$).[14]

2.4 Discussion of Platelet Products in Autologous Fat Grafting

Addition of PRP to autologous fat grafting and lipofilling is another application in plastic surgery. However, publications are conflicting with some showing benefit, some equivalent, and some detrimental.[15,16,17,18,19,20,21,22,23,24,25,26] Faster recovery without significant improvement in graft retention or volume is another reported outcome. Despite employing almost routine autologous fat grafting as an adjunct to other facial procedures for 15 years, we have generally not added PRP to our aliquots, since early attempts using the AdiPrep II system over a 1-year timeframe produced less than expected fat graft retention. Studies suggest that the inflammation included in some PRP solutions may be counterproductive or overcome the benefits from augmented levels of endothelial and vascular growth factors.[27] Some preparatory systems limit nonplatelet cell lines more than others, and the concentration of granulocytes and erythrocytes may be equally, if not more, important than platelets, especially in delicate tissue such as adipose where retention rates already vary widely.

The unpredictable results seen here and in published studies may result from variability in the purity of PRP. For example, the AdiPrep II was inconsistent in our experience in limiting the buffy coat or red blood cells. It has been shown that different systems for PRP production produce different admixtures and concentrations.[14] We have noticed variation in clarity of the plasma-containing platelets between the three systems in our practice: Adi-Prep II; PurePRP (EmCyte Corporation; Fort Myers, FL); and EclipsePRP (Eclipse Aesthetics LLC; The Colony, TX).

2.5 Conclusion

While PRP has been shown to be useful in a variety of settings for aesthetic facial surgery including treatment of rhytids, atrophic acne scars, androgenic alopecia, and as an additive to autologous fat grafting,[15,16,17,18,19] we have found its greatest benefit as a promoter of wound healing and as a fibrin sealant intraoperatively. With the pressure of rapid and efficient recovery as a constant patient concern, any treatment to accelerate recovery is welcome.

References

[1] Man D, Plosker H, Winland-Brown JE. The use of autologous platelet-rich plasma (platelet gel) and autologous platelet-poor plasma (fibrin glue) in cosmetic surgery. Plast Reconstr Surg. 2001; 107(1):229–237, discussion 238–239
[2] Kang RS, Lee MK, Seth R, Keller GS. Platelet-rich plasma in cosmetic surgery. Otorhinolaryngology Clinics Int J. 2013; 5(1):24–28
[3] Eppley BL, Pietrzak WS, Blanton M. Platelet-rich plasma: a review of biology and applications in plastic surgery. Plast Reconstr Surg. 2006; 118(6):147e–159e
[4] Personal observation at the University of Michigan, Department of Dermatology, as a plastic surgery resident, 1979
[5] Ellis DA, Shaikh A. The ideal tissue adhesive in facial plastic and reconstructive surgery. J Otolaryngol. 1990; 19(1):68–72
[6] Marchac D, Sándor G. Face lifts and sprayed fibrin glue: an outcome analysis of 200 patients. Br J Plast Surg. 1994; 47(5):306–309
[7] Marchac D, Greensmith AL. Early postoperative efficacy of fibrin glue in face lifts: a prospective randomized trial. Plast Reconstr Surg. 2005; 115(3):911–916, discussion 917–918
[8] Gruber RG, Zeidler KR, Berkowitz RL. Desmopressin as a hemostatic agent to provide a dry intraoperative field in rhinoplasty. Plast Reconstr Surg. 2015; 135(5):1337–1340
[9] Berkowitz RL, Zeidler KR. Reducing or eliminating ecchymoses in rhinoplasty as presented to the Rhinoplasty Society. April 2015; San Francisco, CA
[10] Berkowitz RL, Gruber RG. Management of the nasal dorsum: construction and maintenance of a Barrel Vault. Clin Plast Surg. 2016; 43(1):59–72
[11] Zoumalan R, Rizk SS. Hematoma rates in drainless deep-plane face-lift surgery with and without the use of fibrin glue. Arch Facial Plast Surg. 2008; 10(2):103–107
[12] Grover R, Jones BM, Waterhouse N. The prevention of haematoma following rhytidectomy: a review of 1078 consecutive facelifts. Br J Plast Surg. 2001; 54(6):481–486
[13] Kamer FM, Song AU. Hematoma formation in deep plane rhytidectomy. Arch Facial Plast Surg. 2000; 2(4):240–242
[14] Giordano S, Koskivuo I, Suominen E, Veräjänkorva E. Tissue sealants may reduce haematoma and complications in facelifts: a meta-analysis of comparative studies. J Plast Reconstr Aesthet Surg. 2017; 70(3):297–306
[15] Motosko CC, Khouri KS, Poudrier G, Sinno S, Hazen A. Evaluating platelet rich therapy for facial aesthetics and alopecia: a critical review of the literature. Plast Reconstr Surg. 2018; 141(5):1115–1123
[16] Cervelli V, Palla L, Pascali M, De Angelis B, Curcio BC, Gentile P. Autologous platelet-rich plasma mixed with purified fat graft in aesthetic plastic surgery. Aesthetic Plast Surg. 2009; 33(5):716–721
[17] Fontdevila J, Guisantes E, Martínez E, Prades E, Berenguer J. Double-blind clinical trial to compare autologous fat grafts versus autologous fat grafts with PDGF: no effect of PDGF. Plast Reconstr Surg. 2014; 134(2):219e–230e
[18] Frautschi RS, Hashem AM, Halasa B, Cakmakoglu C, Zins JE. Current evidence for clinical efficacy of platelet rich plasma in aesthetic surgery: a systematic review. Aesthet Surg J. 2017; 37(3):353–362
[19] Layliev J, Gupta V, Kaoutzanis C, et al. Incidence and preoperative risks for major complications in aesthetic rhinoplasty: analysis of 4978 patients. Aesthet Surg J. 2017; 37(7):757–767
[20] Gentile P, De Angelis B, Pasin M, et al. Adipose-derived stromal vascular fraction cells and platelet-rich plasma: basic

and clinical evaluation for cell-based therapies in patients with scars on the face. J Craniofac Surg. 2014; 25(1):267–272

[21] Willemsen JC, van der Lei B, Vermeulen KM, Stevens HP. The effects of platelet-rich plasma on recovery time and aesthetic outcome in facial rejuvenation: preliminary retrospective observations. Aesthetic Plast Surg. 2014; 38(5): 1057–1063

[22] Willemsen JCN, Van Dongen J, Spiekman M, et al. The additional of platelet rich plasm to facial lipofilling: a double-blind, placebo-controlled randomized trial. Plast Reconstr Surg. 2018; 141(2):331–343

[23] Fontdevila J, Guisantes E, Martínez E, Prades E, Berenguer J. Double-blind clinical trial to compare autologous fat grafts versus autologous fat grafts with PDGF: no effect of PDGF. Plast Reconstr Surg. 2014; 134(2):219e–230e

[24] Keyhan SO, Hemmat S, Badri AA, Abdeshahzadeh A, Khiabani K. Use of platelet-rich fibrin and platelet-rich plasma in combination with fat graft: which is more effective during facial lipostructure? J Oral Maxillofac Surg. 2013; 71(3):610–621

[25] Cervelli V, Palla L, Pascali M, De Angelis B, Curcio BC, Gentile P. Autologous platelet-rich plasma mixed with purified fat graft in aesthetic plastic surgery. Aesthetic Plast Surg. 2009; 33(5): 716–721

[26] Cervelli V, Nicoli F, Spallone D, et al. Treatment of traumatic scars using fat grafts mixed with platelet-rich plasma, and resurfacing of skin with the 1540 nm nonablative laser. Clin Exp Dermatol. 2012; 37(1):55–61

[27] Cervelli V, Gentile P, Scioli MG, et al. Application of platelet-rich plasma in plastic surgery: clinical and in vitro evaluation. Tissue Eng Part C Methods. 2009; 15(4):625–634

3
Platelet-Rich Plasma for Rejuvenation and Augmentation

Jeanette M. Black and Lisa M. Donofrio

Abstract

Platelets contain α-granules, which release growth factors that stimulate collagen synthesis and aid in wound healing. This mechanism makes platelet-rich plasma (PRP) an appealing treatment modality for rejuvenation and augmentation. PRP has been used for the improvement of skin laxity, rhytides, and periocular rejuvenation. Additionally, PRP has been combined with other treatment modalities aimed at rejuvenation and augmentation such as microneedling, laser resurfacing, fat grafting, and hyaluronic acid filler injections to improve the recovery and outcomes of these procedures. Various preparations of PRP including a variant called platelet-rich fibrin matrix have been used for rejuvenation. It is difficult to interpret current studies utilizing PRP for aesthetic purposes due to lack of standardized preparation techniques and delivery modalities. Even though substantial objective evidence-based data is lacking, PRP seems to be safe, demonstrates high patient satisfaction, and remains a promising treatment option for aesthetics. Future studies are warranted to determine the optimal PRP preparation techniques and treatment protocols.

Keywords: PRP, platelet-rich plasma, rejuvenation, augmentation, growth factors, rhytides, collagen, fat grafting, periocular rejuvenation

Key Points

- Platelets secret growth factors that increase collagen synthesis, making platelet-rich plasma (PRP) an appealing treatment modality for rejuvenation and augmentation.
- PRP has been studied for skin rejuvenation and improvement of rhytides.
- PRP has been studied for periocular rejuvenation.
- PRP has been combined with microneedling and laser resurfacing to improve the recovery and outcomes of skin rejuvenation.
- PRP has been combined with hyaluronic acid filler injections and fat grafting to improve the recovery and outcomes of augmentation.
- A variant of PRP called platelet-rich fibrin matrix has been reported to also be effective for skin rejuvenation and improvement of rhytides.
- PRP has been combined with growth factor preparations for potentially increased efficacy.
- Current studies remain difficult to interpret and compare due to lack of standardized PRP preparation techniques and delivery modalities.
- Although current studies lack sufficient objective evidence-based data, PRP appears to be safe and is a promising treatment modality.
- Future studies are warranted to determine how PRP can best be utilized for rejuvenation and augmentation.

3.1 Theory Behind Platelet-Rich Plasma For Rejuvenation And Augmentation

Extrinsic aging of the skin is a result of damage from environmental factors such as ultraviolet (UV) radiation causing epidermal thinning, atypia of keratinocytes, collagen degradation, and reduced skin elasticity.[1] Skin aging is histologically characterized by a flattened dermal–epidermal junction, dermal atrophy, and decreased fibroblasts.[2] These changes manifest clinically as xerosis, atrophy, dyschromia, rhytides, and decreased elasticity.[3] Biostimulating treatments that reverse this damage may potentially obtain more natural looking results, provide a longer duration of correction, prevent future damage, have improved safety profiles, and complement other treatment modalities. Many aesthetic procedures intend to correct aged skin by stimulating a wound healing response to repair such damage. This is often achieved either by implanting a foreign material such as with dermal fillers or by creating microinjuries to the skin in a controlled manner such as with chemical peels, lasers, light devices, microneedling, subcision, radiofrequency, and ultrasound treatments. Implanting foreign materials and purposely injuring the skin is not without risks and limitations. Foreign material implantation may lead to complications including infection, immune reactions, improper placement, migration, nodules, swelling, and vascular occlusions.[4] Excess injury to the skin with chemicals, lasers, microneedling, subcision, radiofrequency, and/or ultrasound is also a risk, and these treatments are limited to avoid such complications.[5] An ideal cosmetic treatment would stimulate a wound healing and repair mechanism without the associated risks of the injury itself. Biostimulation with autologous platelet-rich plasma (PRP) has the potential to reverse the damage seen in aged skin on a molecular level by releasing growth factors designed to repair the damage without the associated risks of other treatment modalities.[2,3] By using autologous blood products, there is no risk associated with foreign materials and a wound healing response can be triggered without actually causing gross injury. Additionally, PRP may be used to augment and enhance recovery from other treatments.[3] In the past decade, PRP has been used either by itself or in combination with other procedures for skin rejuvenation and augmentation.[2,6,7,8]

During normal wound healing, platelets degranulate releasing α-granules, which contain key growth factors needed to stimulate wound healing.[9] These growth factors include platelet-derived growth factor, transforming growth factor, vascular endothelial growth factor, epidermal growth factor, and insulin-like growth factor.[2,7,10] The growth factors are chemotactic for monocytes, fibroblasts, stem cells, endothelial cells, and osteoblasts and are mitogenic for fibroblasts, smooth muscle cells, osteoblasts, endothelial cells, and keratinocytes.[10] Receptors for these growth factors are found on adult mesenchymal stem cells, fibroblasts, osteoblasts, endothelial cells, and epidermal cells.[11] They enhance production of collagen and fibronectin, increase vascular permeability, and promote angiogenisis.[10] PRP is a autologous solution of plasma containing 2 to 10 times the baseline concentration of platelets found in normal human plasma.[3] This supraphysiological concentration of growth factors can be used to accelerate tissue remodeling and regeneration.[12]

PRP also contains fibrin, fibronectin, and vitronectin, which also play an important role in cell migration, attachment, proliferation, differentiation, and extracellular matrix accumulation.[2] PRP has been used to capitalize on the healing process stimulated by platelets on a cellular level.[8] To intrinsically rejuvenate aged skin, this growth factor cascade stimulates fibroblasts and increases the synthesis of collagen and other matrix components used to repair the damaged and degraded extracellular matrix.[2] Such properties of PRP make it an intriguing treatment modality for rejuvenation and augmentation. The U.S. food and Drug Administration (FDA) had cleared commercially available PRP separation systems for use in combination with allograft or autograft bone before implantation and in the case of select systems for the treatment of nonhealing diabetic ulcers.[3] Injection of PRP for indications such as skin rejuvenation and augmentation are currently off FDA labeling.[3]

3.2 PRP for Skin Rejuvenation And Rhytides

Both animal and human models have been used to study the regenerative effects of PRP on the skin. Studies have included many measurements of efficacy including histological evaluation, patient satisfaction scores, wrinkle scores, and various other parameters. Most clinical studies are small, lack control groups, and use inconsistent treatment regimens and outcome measurements, all factors making head-to-head comparison difficult.

Cho et al used a mice model to demonstrate the effects of PRP on photo-aged skin.[1] In the study, 30 mice were irradiated with UVB for 8 weeks and divided into three treatment groups.[1] One treatment group received PRP injections, one saline injections, and one no injections.[1] At 4 weeks after the final treatment, wrinkle analysis showed significantly reduced wrinkles in the PRP group relative to the two.[1] Biopsy specimens revealed significantly increased dermal thickness and in vitro assays demonstrated increased fibroblast proliferation and collagen production in the PRP group.[1]

Histological changes in human skin after PRP corroborate the findings seen in animal models. Abuaf et al evaluated histological changes in infra-auricular skin sampled from 20 patients before and after treatment with PRP injections on the right side and saline injections on the left side.[13] They found a 46% increase in collagen densities in the saline side and 89% increase in the PRP side.[13] This study demonstrates that PRP may increase dermal collagen levels not only by growth factors but also by microinjuries caused by injection needling.[13] Charles-de-Sa et al examined histological changes in 13 patients treated 3 months after a single PRP injection in the mastoid area.[14] Biopsies to demonstrate histologic changes found increased reticular dermal thickening with increased deposition of elastic fibers and collagen.[14]

Cameli et al reported statistically significant improvement in skin texture, gross elasticity, skin smoothness, skin barrier function, and capacitance in 12 patients treated with 3 monthly sessions of PRP.[2] The subjects received intradermal injections to the forehead, crow's feet, cheeks, and nasolabial folds and were evaluated 1 month after their final treatment.[2] Treatments were well tolerated without complication.[2]

Yuksel et al evaluated 10 patients treated with PRP injections to the crow's feet and PRP application post "dermaroller" treatment to forehead, malar, and jaw area.[15] The patients received 3 biweekly treatments were evaluated 3 weeks after their last treatment. They showed statistically significant improvement in skin firmness, sagging, general appearance, and wrinkles with no significant complications reported.[15]

Elnehrawy et al followed 20 patients treated with PRP for facial wrinkles including nasolabial folds, crow's feet, and transverse forehead lines 8 weeks after a single session of intradermal PRP injections.[13] They reported significant correction of wrinkles without any concerning side effects.[13] Interestingly, there was notable improvement of nasolabial folds as compared to the other treatment areas.[13]

Redalelli et al followed 23 patients receiving 3 monthly PRP injections on the face and neck.[16] Dermoscopic, digital, photographic images, patient satisfaction scores, and physician satisfaction scores were taken at baseline and at 4 weeks after the final injection.[16] They reported statistically significant improvement in nasolabial folds, horizontal neck bands, periocular wrinkles, skin microrelief, skin snap test, skin homogeneity and texture, and skin tonicity.[16] None of the participants experienced serious or persistent side effects with the most common adverse effects being bruising, mild erythema, and a burning sensation lasting for a few minutes after the injection.[16] This burning sensation was likely due to calcium chloride which was used as an activator in the PRP preparation.[16]

Mikhael and El-Esawy conducted a 6-month study with 20 patients receiving 3 monthly sessions of PRP injections.[17]

They found improvements in clinical photographs, patient satisfaction questionnaires, and physicians impression scores at 1 month after the final treatment session compared to pretreatment assessments.[17] The procedure was also safe and well tolerated with only transient, mild injection site reactions as side effects.[17]

Using a more robust study design, Gawdat et al performed a split-faced trial of 20 patients randomly assigned to receive PRP injections on one side of their face and mesotherapy with a formulation of "readymade growth factors" on the other.[18] The patients received 6 biweekly sessions and were followed up for 6 months.[18] Both procedures yielded significant improvement in skin turgor, overall vitality, and increased epidermal and dermal thickness.[18] However, the investigators found higher patient satisfaction and increased longevity with more sustained improvement after PRP treatments compared to mesotherapy treatments.[18] This trial is noteworthy because it is one of the few controlled studies with a longer follow-up period and because it included both qualitative clinical outcome measures as well as histologic. Nevertheless, the sample size was small, making sweeping generalizations difficult.

Kamakura et al published a larger prospective study including 2005 patients treated with injections of PRP mixed with a basic fibroblast growth factor into rhytides including nasolabial folds, marionette lines, nasojugal grooves, supraorbital grooves, midcheek grooves, forehead, temple, glabella, perioral, neck, and dorsal hand.[19] The patients received one treatment and were followed up at various points in time for the next 6 months.[19] The time after treatment to show apparent improvements in wrinkles was on average 65.4 days.[19]

Both physicians and patients demonstrated high satisfaction, and the only notable complication was overcorrection, which decreased in incidence over time as the treating clinicians became more familiar with dosing titration and injection techniques. The authors did not compare this combination solution to PRP alone but did mention that in their prior experience, PRP monotherapy was not sufficient for deeper fold correction.[19]

Platelet-rich fibrin matrix (PRFM) is another autologous product most commonly used in oral maxofacial and plastic surgery to minimize hematoma formation. Preparation involves mixing PRP with thrombin to form a hemostatic gel with sustained release of growth factors.[20] This application is discussed further in Chapter 2. Sclafani et al have published several studies using PRFM for treatment of facial rhytides. However, per methodology descriptions, this solution appears to be more akin to PRP that has been activated and allowed to partially polymerize than true PRFM, which is thick and cannot easily be extruded through a syringe (reports using a 30-gauge needle). In his first paper, Sclafani treated 15 patients with intradermal injections of PRFM into the nasolabial folds.[20] He found statistically significant improvement in folds with increasing improvements in wrinkles scores at weeks 2, 6, and maximum improvement at 12 weeks after treatment.[20] No significant adverse events or complications were reported.[20]

Sclafani and McCormick published a report of four patients that received PRFM injections injected to upper arm skin and biopsies were taken prior to treatment and repeated over 10 weeks after the treatment.[21] Histological evaluation revealed evidence of activated fibroblasts and new collagen deposition as early as 7 days after treatment and these changes continued throughout 10 weeks.[21] Development of new blood vessels, intradermal collections of adipocytes, and stimulation of subdermal adipocytes were noted by 19 days.[21] These findings became more pronounced over the duration of the study, although fibroblast response became less pronounced by the end of the study.[21]

Finally, Scalfani performed a chart review of 50 patients treated with PRFM for rhytides and skin rejuvenation with follow-up of at least 3 months.[22] The patients received an average go 1.6 treatments and had an average follow-up interval of 8 months.[22] At follow-up, most patients were satisfied with their results and reported that the treatments were well tolerated.[22] These findings of high patient satisfaction and tolerability with PRFM are consistent with studies using other variants of PRP for similar purposes.[22] Future studies are needed to compare the efficacy, longevity, and tolerability of Scalfani's PRFM as compared to other PRP preparations. Clarification of terminology and standardization of preparation protocols is paramount for the integration and acceptance of PRP in the aesthetic medical field. Without clear definitions, there is confusion among providers who cannot effectively reproduce outcomes reported in clinical trials.

3.3 Platelet-Rich Plasma for Periocular Rejuvenation

Periocular rejuvenation and augmentation has proven to be particularly challenging, and many procedures yield unwanted complications or unsatisfactory results.[4,5]

Complications have included bruising, persistent swelling, nodule formations, vascular occlusions, and even blindness.[4,5] PRP may offer a safer approach to periocular rejuvenation, an important benefit making autologous therapies appealing to clinicians and patients alike.

Mehryan et al followed 10 patients after a single intradermal injection of PRP into the tear trough area and crow's feet.[23] They evaluated the effects on melanin content, color homogeneity, epidermal stratum corneum hydration, and wrinkle volume 3 months after the injection and found statistically significant improvements in infraorbital color.[23] They did not show statistically significant improvements on the other measured parameters but did note improvements in both physician's and patient's satisfaction scores.[23]

Ramaganont et al reported a split-face, randomized double-blind, placebo control study with 20 patients.[24] PRP was injected into crow's feet, and preauricular area of one side of the face and normal saline was injected on the other.[24] Three months after the injections, there were significant reductions in rhytides on both the treatment and placebo sides, but no significant difference between the two treatments, a finding suggesting that the needling associated with injection may have substantial impact on periocular skin.[24] Regardless, patient satisfaction was high with an excellent safety profile.[24]

Kang et al evaluated 20 patients seeking improvement of infraorbital skin tone and wrinkles.[25] Ten patients received PRP on one side of the face and platelet-poor plasma (PPP) on the other side.[25] The other 10 received PRP injections on one side and saline injections on the other.[25] Patients received 3 monthly infraorbital treatment sessions.[25] Outcomes measures included self-assessment questionnaires, subjective satisfaction scores, and clinical assessment by three blinded dermatologists who compared photographs obtained at baseline and at 3 months after the final treatment.[25] Infraorbital skin treated with PRP showed significant improvement in wrinkles and skin tone compared with PPP or saline treated skin.[25]

Nofal et al followed 30 patients treated with PRP for improvement of periorbital pigmentation.[26] Patients were treated with 7 biweekly intradermal injections of PRP on the left periorbital area and 7 weekly carboxytherapy to the right periorbital areas.[26] They found that PRP and carboxytherapy were relatively comparable in their efficacy for the treatment of periorbital hyperpigmentation.[26] The authors reported that side effects such as bruising and pain were more common in the PRP treated side as compared to the side treated with carboxytherapy.[26] Given PRP's impressive tolerability and safety profile, it continues to be a particularly intriguing treatment option for periocular rejuvenation.

3.4 Platelet-Rich Plasma with Microneedling and Laser Resurfacing for Skin Rejuvenation

The combination of PRP with other aesthetic procedures intended for skin rejuvenation could potentially afford many benefits. As mentioned above, some of the benefits from PRP may be attributed to the act of injection needling itself.

Additionally, given the penetration of PRP applied to skin with a compromised epidermal barrier, PRP application to skin after microneedling and laser resurfacing has been used to potentially enhance the outcomes of and speed recovery from these procedures.[27,28,29]

Na et al evaluated 25 patients treated with fractional carbon dioxide (CO_2) laser on the bilateral inner arm.[27] After the laser treatment, PRP was applied to one arm and normal saline to the other, then patients were followed up for 28 days.[27] The investigators found a significant decrease in both melanin and erythema indices as well as a faster recovery of transepidermal water loss on the side treated with PRP.[27] Skin biopsies taken from five patients showed thicker collagen bundles on the PRP treated side.[27] These findings suggest that the application of PRP may be an effective method to enhance wound healing, reduce transient unwanted adverse effects, and improve skin tightening after laser resurfacing.[27]

Shin et al followed 22 patients treated with three sessions of laser treatments.[28] Eleven of the women had PRP applied after their procedure and the other 11 did not.[28] Satisfaction ratings for improvement in skin texture and fine wrinkles were 100% in the group treated with PRP plus fractional CO_2 laser versus 58% in the group treated with fractional CO_2 laser alone.[28] At 1-month posttreatment, the erythema index decreased significantly in the PRP group, and biopsy specimens from the PRP treated skin showed increased collagen, higher numbers of fibroblasts, and longer length of the dermoepidermal junction.[28]

Similar to combining PRP with laser resurfacing, combination PRP plus microneedling has become an increasingly popular procedure. And there is a growing body of literature investigating the effects of microneedling with and without application of PRP for many indications.[29] A more in-depth discussion of these procedures can be found in Chapters 6 and 9. Briefly, it is likely that adding PRP to microneedling procedures aimed at skin rejuvenation improves outcomes and helps to minimize transient side effects as is seen when PRP is combined with laser resurfacing.[29] Sasaki used fluorescein-labeled platelets to attempt to further understand how PRP penetrates after microneedling procedures.[30] He used confocal laser microscopy to measure the absorption of PRP and determined that the optimal time for massaging PRP down 1.0 mm microneedling channels was between 5 to 30 minutes after microneedling.[30] Future studies need to done to further analyze how PRP penetrates the skin with application during both microneedling and laser resurfacing procedures.

3.5 Platelet-Rich Plasma Combined with Fat Grafting and Hyaluronic Acid Injections for Enhanced Augmentation

Combining PRP with other injectable substances such as autologous fat or hyaluronic acid filler is appealing, since the combination may provide synergistic effects. Augmentation with fat grafting and hyaluronic acid fillers offer impressive aesthetic results, but these treatments have risks of adverse reactions and/or lack longevity.[4] The addition of PRP may potentially decrease the volume needed for sustained correction, provide a scaffold for delayed biostimulation that increases longevity of temporary fillers, aid in engraftment of autologous fat, and help limit potential complications.

Ulusal published a series of 94 patients treated with intradermal injections of PRP combined with hyaluronic acid.[31] He found high patient satisfaction and a statistically significant improvement in skin firmness-sagging, skin texture, and general appearance based on ratings by three independent physicians as well as the patients themselves.[31] There were no significant complications reported.[31]

Another study involved 31 patients treated with hyaluronic acid mixed with PRP delivered via injections and with a "skinroller."[32] Subjects received 3 monthly treatments with outcomes assessed for 6 months after the final session.[32] When compared to baseline, patients demonstrated statistically significant improvement in skin firmness and elasticity and reported no serious complications.[32] Future controlled trials are necessary to compare the efficacy and safety of combination hyaluronic acid and PRP versus each product separately. It is imperative that these studies explicit outline the preparation protocols and final solution composition, as small changes in platelet, leukocyte, and erythrocyte concentration and dose may impact how the solutions interact and synergize. Application techniques, whether administered by injection or more superficially through microneedling pores, must also be examined rigorously.

The evidence for combining PRP with autologous fat grafting is controversial with some reports suggesting increased graft survival and hemostasis and others not. See Chapter 1 for a more in depth discussion. In short, Wellemsen et al reported a retrospective analysis of 82 patients with regard to recovery time and the aesthetic improvement treatment with fat grafting and minimal access cranial suspension (MACS)-lift with and without the addition of PRP.[33] Adding PRP to facial lipofilling reduced recovery time and improved the overall aesthetic outcome of a MACS-lift.[33] A randomized clinical trial by Fontdevila and colleagues found no difference in bilateral volume gain or maintenance via computed tomography imaging of grafts plus PRP versus grafts only, whereas two other blinded clinical trials looking different combination therapies did report benefits.[34,35,36,37,38] These differences may result from the diverse composition and preparation of PRP solutions. Inclusion of the buffy coat may have substantial impact on autologous fat graft survival due to inflammatory effects. So, like other PRP combinations, larger controlled trials with explicitly outlined, standardized techniques are still needed.

3.6 Techniques and Considerations

Although PRP has been utilized for over four decades in orthopedics, maxillofacial and other surgical fields of medicine, it has been adopted only more recently for aesthetic purposes, likely due to insufficient, small scale, or conflicting literature without clear objective evidence regarding its efficacy.[39,40] Many systemic reviews have been conducted regarding the use of PRP for rejuvenation and augmentation.[39,40,41] In 2017, Frautschi et al published a comprehensive review searching for reports of PRP in aesthetic medicine published from 1950 to 2015.[39] After review of 38 reports, the authors concluded that the published studies produced promising, context-dependent results but lacked consistent reporting of preparation, composition, and activation methods, making any meaningful meta-analysis unrealistic. Moreover, the majority of studies were case series lacking controls and while most studies claimed effectiveness, objective measures were only used in 47% of the studies.[39] A review of studies on PRP in aesthetics from 2006 to 2015 by Motosko et al agreed that, although the majority of studies yield positive results and are safe, there is significant variation in preparation and treatment protocols, which makes conclusive findings difficult.[40] More rigorously designed studies for acne scarring, including randomized controlled and split face trials as well as flow cytometry reports, have been published since that time and lend further credence to this potential rejuvenate modality.[2,42,43,44,45]

Because PRP is autologous, there is innate variability in PRP platelet concentration.[46] Platelet concentrations in humans can range from 150,000 to 450,000/µl, so this variation can potentially impact PRP concentration by three-fold.[39] Most of the current studies do not account for baseline platelet levels or report the platelet concentration of PRP. There is also discussion whether concentration versus total absolute platelet dose/count may be better metrics to measure efficacy, since the latter is not volume dependent.[39] These studies also fail to account for the effect of various common pharmaceutical agents potentially affecting platelet function (i.e., aspirin, statins, antibiotics, and serotonin reuptake inhibitors), though a single small study suggests these medications may have little impact.[33]

Another topic of much debate and perhaps equally important to platelet concentration/count is the inclusion or exclusion of other cell lines. Leukocytes and erythrocytes can substantially impact PRP's activity and growth factor profile. Studies of high platelet-, high leukocyte-producing PRP systems report increased concentrations of many catabolic molecules.[47] White blood cells found in the buffy coat produce a large amounts of matrix metalloproteinases,[48] which may limit tissue repair and degrade extracellular matrix, as seen in photoaging.[49] Red blood cells release reactive oxygen species, alter solution pH, and may deposit hemosiderin,[47] all factor that can influence tissue response and resultant outcomes. Understanding the effects on PRP of these cell lines for each of the different aesthetic indications is critical to the adoption and standardization of such treatments.[47,48,49]

The methods of PRP preparation remain variable and often poorly described, thus studies are difficult to interpret, replicate, or compare head-to-head.[50] PRP preparation methodology warrants increased attention.[38] In the authors' opinion PRP preparation protocols must be better classified and standardized before expanding on the current literature and evaluating clinical outcomes. At a minimum, future studies should report clear preparation methods along with the starting and final cellular compositions of their therapeutic solutions. Frautschi et al recommended a classification system that can be used to help produce scientifically grounded conclusions and help facilitate a clearer understanding of situations in which PRP is most effective.[39] The proposed FIT PAW classification system includes seven components: (1) force of centrifugation, (2) sequence of centrifugation, (3) time of centrifugation, (4) platelet concentration, (5) anticoagulant use, (6) activator use, and (7) white blood cell composition.[39] The use of a reporting system such as this may help demystify PRP and allow for consistent results across different medical specialties and treatment sites, all prerequisites to the development of well-founded PRP applications in aesthetics.[39]

Despite these limitations, reported methods of using PRP for rejuvenation and augmentation include: cutaneous injections, saturation with microneedling (▶ Fig. 3.1, ▶ Fig. 3.2, ▶ Fig. 3.3, ▶ Fig. 3.4) and laser resurfacing, as well as combination with fat grafting and injectable fillers.[34] PRP is commonly injected intradermally (▶ Fig. 3.5, ▶ Fig. 3.6, ▶ Fig. 3.7) and most cases in the literature report minimal complications with this method. There were reports of transient bruising and pain with periorbital intradermal injections of PRP.[26] One of the authors (J.B.) prefers to use a cannula for periorbital PRP injections (▶ Fig. 3.8) finding that this technique minimizes the incidence and severity of swelling and bruising, but acknowledging that it prohibits the plane of intradermal injection. PRP has been prepared with other active ingredients such as growth factor formulations and as discussed above, with autologous fat, and hyaluronic acid fillers.[17,31,39] The implications of such combinations are unclear, but the potential for synergistic outcome remains alluring. Further studies are needed to evaluate how combinations and delivery methods can be optimized to achieve the most effective outcomes.

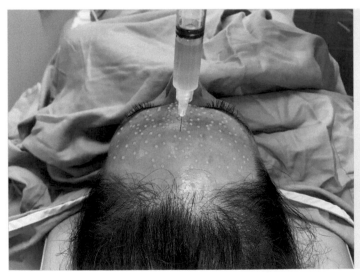

Fig. 3.1 PRP applied topically prior to microneedling.

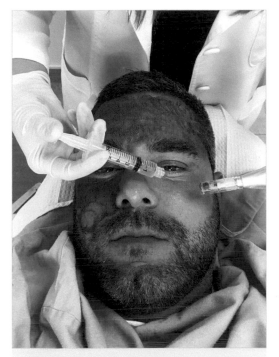

Fig. 3.2 PRP applied topically in combination with microneedling.

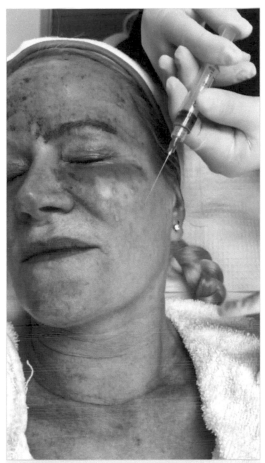

Fig. 3.4 PRP applied topically in combination with microneedling.

Fig. 3.3 PRP applied topically in combination with microneedling.

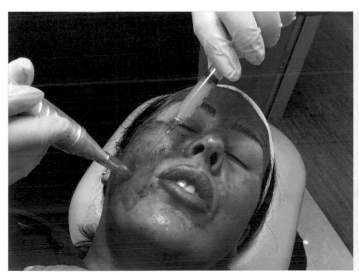

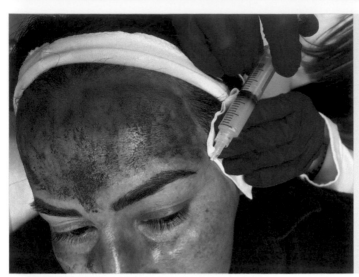

Fig. 3.5 PRP injected intradermally with a needle to the periorbital area.

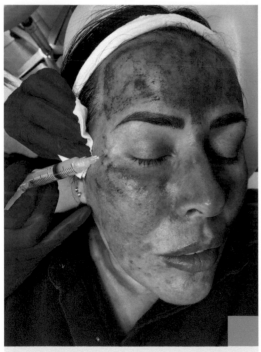

Fig. 3.6 PRP injected intradermally with a needle to the periorbital area.

Although current studies are limited and objective data is lacking, the current literature demonstrates compelling evidence of histological and image-based efficacy, high patient and physician satisfaction, impressive tolerability and safety profiles, and promising proof of concept. It is obvious that there is great potential for the role of PRP in the future of aesthetics both by itself and in combination with other types of procedures. Nevertheless, at this time, prospective, randomized, controlled trials with adequate power are required to raise the level of evidence to a higher level. In the authors' personal experience using PRP in clinical practice and in clinical trials, the treatment has been cost effective, safe, and complements other procedures such as fat grafting, injectable fillers, microneedling, and ablative laser resurfacing.

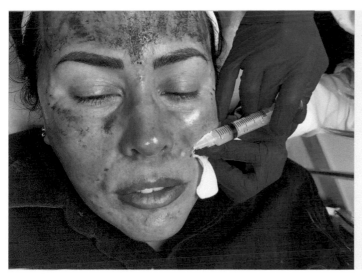
Fig. 3.7 PRP injected intradermally with a needle to the nasolabial area.

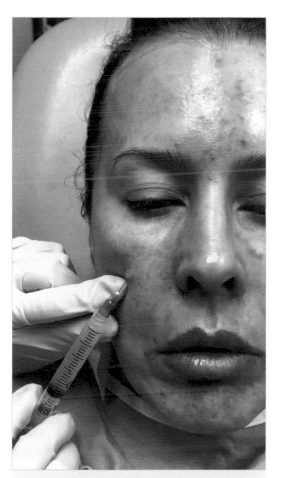
Fig. 3.8 PRP injected subdermally with a cannula to the infraorbital area.

References

[1] Cho JM, Lee YH, Baek RM, Lee SW. Effect of platelet-rich plasma on ultraviolet b-induced skin wrinkles in nude mice. J Plast Reconstr Aesthet Surg. 2011; 64(2):e31–e39

[2] Cameli N, Mariano M, Cordone I, Abril E, Masi S, Foddai ML. Autologous pure platelet-rich plasma dermal injections for facial skin rejuvenation: clinical, instrumental, and flow cytometry assessment. Dermatol Surg. 2017; 43 (6):826–835

[3] Fabi S, Sundaram H. The potential of topical and injectable growth factors and cytokines for skin rejuvenation. Facial Plast Surg. 2014; 30(2):157–171

[4] Vanaman M, Fabi SG, Carruthers J. Complications in the cosmetic patient: a review and our experience (Part 1). Dermatol Surg. 2016; 42(1):1–11

[5] Vanaman M, Fabi SG, Carruthers J. Complication in the cosmetic patient: a review and our experience (Part 2). Dermatol Surg. 2016; 42(1):12–20

[6] Moioli EK, Bolotin D, Alam M. Regenerative medicine and stem cells in dermatology. Dermatol Surg. 2017; 43(5):625–634

[7] Elghblawi E. Platelet-rich plasma, the ultimate secret for youthful skin elixir and hair growth triggering. J of Cos Derm. 2018; 17(3):423–430

[8] Leo MS, Kumar AS, Kirit R, Konathan R, Sivamani RK. Systematic review of the use of platelet-rich plasma in aesthetic dermatology. J Cosmet Dermatol. 2015; 14(4):315–323

[9] Lubkowska A, Dolegowska B, Banfi G. Growth factor content in PRP and their applicability in medicine. J Biol Regul Homeost Agents. 2012; 26(2) Suppl 1:3S–22S

[10] Sclafani AP, Azzi J. Platelet preparations for use in facial rejuvenation and wound healing: a critical review of current literature. Aesthetic Plast Surg. 2015; 39(4):495–505

[11] Marx RE. Platelet-rich plasma: evidence to support its use. J Oral Maxillofac Surg. 2004; 62(4):489–496

[12] Elnehrawy NY, Ibrahim ZA, Eltoukhy AM, Nagy HM. Assessment of the efficacy and safety of single platelet-rich plasma injection on different types and grades of facial wrinkles. J Cosmet Dermatol. 2017; 16(1):103–111

[13] Abuaf OK, Yildiz H, Baloglu H, Bilgili ME, Simsek HA, Dogan B. Histologic evidence of new collagen formation using

platelet-rich plasma in skin rejuvenation: a prospective controlled clinical study. Ann Dermatol. 2016; 28(6):718–724

[14] Charles-de-Sa L, Gontijo-de-Amorim NF, Takiya CM, et al. Effect of use of platelet-rich plasma (PRP) in skin with intrinsic aging process. Aes Surg Journal. 2018; 38(3):321–328

[15] Yuksel EP, Sahin G, Aydin F, Senturk N, Turanli AY. Evaluation of effects of platelet-rich plasma on human facial skin. J Cosmet Laser Ther. 2014; 16(5):206–208

[16] Redaelli A, Romano D, Marcianó A. Face and neck revitalization with platelet-rich plasma (PRP): clinical outcome in a series of 23 consecutively treated patients. J Drugs Dermatol. 2010; 9(5):466–472

[17] Mikhael NW, El-Esawy FM. Skin rejuvenation with autologous concentrated platelet-rich plasma. Egyptian J Derm and Venerol. 2014; 34(1):5–9

[18] Gawdat HI, Tawdy AM, Hegazy RA, Zakaria MM, Allam RS. Autologous platelet-rich plasma versus readymade growth factors in skin rejuvenation: A split face study. J Cosmet Dermatol. 2017; 16(2):258–264

[19] Kamakura T, Kataoka J, Maeda K, et al. Platelet-rich plasma with basic fibroblast growth factor for treatment of wrinkles and depressed areas of the skin. Plast Reconstr Surg. 2015; 136(5):931–939

[20] Sclafani AP. Platelet-rich fibrin matrix for improvement of deep nasolabial folds. J Cosmet Dermatol. 2010; 9(1):66–71

[21] Sclafani AP, McCormick SA. Induction of dermal collagenesis, angiogenesis, and adipogenesis in human skin by injection of platelet-rich fibrin matrix. Arch Facial Plast Surg. 2012; 14(2):132–136

[22] Sclafani AP. Safety, efficacy, and utility of platelet-rich fibrin matrix in facial plastic surgery. Arch Facial Plast Surg. 2011; 13(4):247–251

[23] Mehryan P, Zartab H, Rajabi A, Pazhoohi N, Firooz A. Assessment of efficacy of platelet-rich plasma (PRP) on infraorbital dark circles and crow's feet wrinkles. J Cosmet Dermatol. 2014; 13(1):72–78

[24] Ramaganont K, Chuanchaiyakul S, Udompataikul M. effect of platelet-rich plasma intradermal injection on the reduction of facial cutaneous wrinkles. Wachira Wechasan.. 2011; 55:9–18

[25] Kang BK, Shin MK, Lee JH, Kim NI. Effects of platelet-rich plasma on wrinkles and skin tone in Asian lower eyelid skin: preliminary results from a prospective, randomised, split-face trial. Eur J Dermatol. 2014; 24(1):100–101

[26] Nofal E, Elkot R, Nofal A, Eldesoky F, Shehata S, Sami M. Evaluation of carboxytherapy and platelet-rich plasma in treatment of periorbital hyperpigmentation: a comparative clinical trial. J Cosmet Dermatol. 2018; •••:1–8

[27] Na JI, Choi JW, Choi HR, et al. Rapid healing and reduced erythema after ablative fractional carbon dioxide laser resurfacing combined with the application of autologous platelet-rich plasma. Dermatol Surg. 2011; 37(4):463–468

[28] Shin MK, Lee JH, Lee SJ, Kim NI. Platelet-rich plasma combined with fractional laser therapy for skin rejuvenation. Dermatol Surg. 2012; 38(4):623–630

[29] Hashim PW, Levy Z, Cohen JL, Goldenberg G. Microneedling therapy with and without platelet-rich plasma. Cutis. 2017; 99(4):239–242

[30] Sasaki GH. Micro-needling depth penetration, presence of pigment particles, and fluorescein-stained plateelts:

clnicial usage for aesthetic concerns. Aesthet Surg J. 2017; 37(1):71–83

[31] Ulusal BG. Platelet-rich plasma and hyaluronic acid - an efficient biostimulation method for face rejuvenation. J Cosmet Dermatol. 2017; 16(1):112–119

[32] Hersant B, SidAhmed-Mezi M, Niddam J, et al. Efficacy of autologous platelet-rich plasma combined with hyaluronic acid on skin facial rejuvenation: a prospective study. J Am Acad Dermatol. 2017; 77(3):584–586

[33] Willemsen JC, van der Lei B, Vermeulen KM, Stevens HP. The effects of platelet-rich plasma on recovery time and aesthetic outcome in facial rejuvenation: preliminary retrospective observations. Aesthetic Plast Surg. 2014; 38(5):1057–1063

[34] Fontdevila J, Guisantes E, Martínez E, Prades E, Berenguer J. Double-blind clinical trial to compare autologous fat grafts versus autologous fat grafts with PDGF: no effect of PDGF. Plast Reconstr Surg. 2014; 134(2):219e–230e

[35] Keyhan SO, Hemmat S, Badri AA, Abdeshahzadeh A, Khiabani K. Use of platelet-rich fibrin and platelet-rich plasma in combination with fat graft: which is more effective during facial lipostructure? J Oral Maxillofac Surg. 2013; 71(3):610–621

[36] Cervelli V, Palla L, Pascali M, De Angelis B, Curcio BC, Gentile P. Autologous platelet-rich plasma mixed with purified fat graft in aesthetic plastic surgery. Aesthetic Plast Surg. 2009; 33(5):716–721

[37] Cervelli V, Nicoli F, Spallone D, et al. Treatment of traumatic scars using fat grafts mixed with platelet-rich plasma, and resurfacing of skin with the 1540 nm nonablative laser. Clin Exp Dermatol. 2012; 37(1):55–61

[38] Cervelli V, Gentile P, Scioli MG, et al. Application of platelet-rich plasma in plastic surgery: clinical and in vitro evaluation. Tissue Eng Part C Methods. 2009; 15(4):625–634

[39] Frautschi RS, Hashem AM, Halasa B, Cakmakoglu C, Zins JE. Current evidence for clinical efficacy of platelet rich plasma in aesthetic surgery: a systemic review. Aesthet Surg J. 2017; 37(3):353–362

[40] Motosko CC, Khouri KS, Poudrier G, Sinno S, Hazen A. Evaluating platelet-rich therapy for facial aesthetics and alopecia: a critical review of the literature. Plast Reconstr Surg. 2018; 141(5):1115–1123

[41] Amini F, Abiri F, Ramasamy TS, Tan ES. Efficacy of platelet rich plasma (PRP) on skin rejuvenation: a systemic review. Iranian J of Derm. 2015; 18(3):119–127

[42] Willemsen JCN, Van Dongen J, Spiekman M, et al. The addition of platelet-rich plasma to facial lipofilling: a double-blinded, placebo-controlled, randomized trial. Plast Reconstr Surg. 2018; 141(2):331–343

[43] Min S, Yoon JY, Park SY, Moon J, Kwon HH, Suh DH. Combination of platelet rich plasma in fractional carbon dioxide laser treatment increased clinical efficacy of for acne scar by enhancement of collagen production and modulation of laser-induced inflammation. Lasers Surg Med. 2018; 50(4):302–310

[44] Ibrahim ZA, El-Ashmawy AA, Shora OA. Therapeutic effect of microneedling and autologous platelet-rich plasma in the treatment of atrophic scars: a randomized study. J Cosmet Dermatol. 2017; 16(3):388–399

[45] Ibrahim MK, Ibrahim SM, Salem AM. Skin microneedling plus platelet-rich plasma versus skin microneedling alone in the

treatment of atrophic post acne scars: a split face comparative study. J Dermatolog Treat. 2018, 29(3):281–286

[46] Weibrich G, Kleis WK, Hafner G, Hitzler WE. Growth factor levels in platelet-rich plasma and correlations with donor age, sex, and platelet count. J Craniomaxillofac Surg. 2002; 30(2):97–102

[47] Magalon J, Bausset O, Serratrice N, et al. Characterization and comparison of 5 platelet-rich plasma preparations in a single-donor model. Arthroscopy. 2014; 30(5):629–638

[48] Oh JH, Kim W, Park KU, Roh YH. Comparison of the cellular composition and cytokine-release kinetics of various platelet-rich plasma preparations. Am J Sports Med. 2015; 43(12):3062–3070

[49] Braun HJ, Kim HJ, Chu CR, Dragoo JL. The effect of platelet-rich plasma formulations and blood products on human synoviocytes: implications for intra-articular injury and therapy. Am J Sports Med. 2014; 42(5):1204–1210

[50] Dhurat R, Sukesh M. Principles and methods of preparation of platelet-rich plasma: a review and author's perspective. J Cutan Aesthet Surg. 2014; 7(4):189–197

4

Platelet-Rich Plasma for Alopecia and Hair Restoration

Jeffrey A. Rapaport, Sarah G. Versteeg, and Aditya K. Gupta

Abstract

Platelet-rich plasma (PRP) therapy is a promising nonsurgical option for alopecia conditions, such as androgenetic alopecia (AGA) and to a less studied extent, alopecia areata (AA) and cicatricial alopecia (CA), with minimal side effects reported. A recent meta-analysis concluded that PRP treatments can achieve treatment success in AGA patients, using hair density as the unit of measure. Improvements in hair count, hair thickness, and microscopic evaluations have also been noted in PRP-treated patients with AGA. PRP may be more successful than other off-label options for the treatment of AA, with the potential to achieve desired results in a shorter timeframe. It may also be of value in treating CA, a rare scarring alopecia condition, as PRP can elicit regenerative pathways. However, the evidence supporting PRP as a treatment for CA is limited, with only case studies published thus far. Combining PRP with surgical hair restoration techniques can result in increased hair growth as PRP can encourage hair grafts to enter the anagen phase. Combining PRP with extracellular matrix (ECM) materials could be beneficial as ECM materials can improve wound healing and donor scarring. To achieve optimum results, it is suggested that PRP should be performed once a month for three months with a platelet concentration of 4 to 7 times the patient's circulating whole blood plate-let levels. Research conducted using randomized controlled trials with long-term follow-up (i.e., 12 months) are required in order to standardize PRP protocols and better quantify antici-pated efficacy.

Keywords: platelet-rich plasma, androgenetic alopecia, alopecia areata, cicatricial alopecia, hair restoration

Key Points

Platelet-rich plasma (PRP) for androgenetic alopecia (AGA)
- Meta-analyses and systematic reviews suggest PRP can improve hair density in AGA patients.

PRP for alopecia areata (AA)
- PRP is a potential option for AA patients. Randomized clinical trials found PRP superior to intralesional triamcinolone acetonide and to minoxidil, but the literature is scant and needs to be replicated.

PRP for cicatricial alopecia (CA)
- No randomized, large-scale PRP studies have been conducted in scarring alopecia patients. Only cases series exist to date, thus the success of PRP to treat CA has not been fully investigated.

PRP with surgical hair restoration
- PRP can be advantageous in surgical hair restoration procedures as activated platelets can promote tissue repair, minimize scarring, and encourage hair growth.

4.1 Introduction

Platelet-rich plasma (PRP) therapy is a promising nonsurgical option for patients suffering from certain types of alopecia. PRP can provide an alternative option for hair loss patients who are not ideal candidates for traditional treatments and can help avoid commonly reported side effects of other available therapies (e.g., skin irritation and sexual dysfunction).[1,2,3,4,5,6] The majority of current evidence explores PRP for management of androgenetic alopecia (AGA) with less data suggesting its use in alopecia areata (AA) and some cicatricial alopecia (CA).

PRP therapy can encourage hair growth through the activity of secreted growth factors and cytokines such as platelet-derived growth factor (PDGF), epidermal growth factor (EGF), and vascular endo-thelial growth factor (VEGF).[7,8,9] Growth factors encourage hair follicles to enter into the then prolong the anagen phase by promoting cell survival, cell proliferation, and angiogenesis through the protein kinase B pathway, inhibition of glycogen synthase kinase 3-β and the degradation of β-catenin (► Fig. 4.1).[7,10] PRP can also help decrease inflammation, prevent follicles from prematurely entering the catagen phase, activate proinflammatory signaling pathways, and impact muscle and fat cells.[11,12,13,14]

4.2 PRP for Androgenetic Alopecia

Androgenetic alopecia (AGA) is the most common type of hair loss, characterized by a hair follicles miniaturization, possibly due to increased levels of dihydrotestosterone (DHT) and/or alterations in the androgen receptor gene.[15,16,17] These progressive follicular changes lead to a decreased number of hairs in the anagen phase, such that terminal follicles convert into vellus-like follicles.[18] PRP can enhance the limited action of growth factors created by increased DHT levels commonly

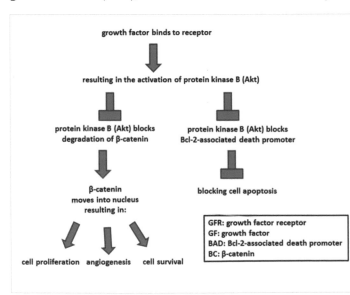

Fig. 4.1 The impact of growth factors on dermal papilla cells. (Adapted from Gupta AK Carviel J. A Mechanistic Model of Platelet-Rich Plasma Treatment for Androgenetic Alopecia. Dermatol Surg Off Publ Am Soc Dermatol Surg Al. 2016;42(12): 1335–1339 and Li ZJ, Choi H-I, Choi D-K, Sohn K-C, Im M, Seo Y-J, et al. Autologous platelet-rich plasma: a potential therapeutic tool for promoting hair growth. Dermatol Surg Off Publ Am Soc Dermatol Surg Al. 2012 Jul;38(7 Pt 1):1040–6.)

associated with AGA.[7] The anti-inflammatory effects of PRP could also be advantageous as dermal inflammatory infiltrates and follicular inflammation have been associated with AGA patients.[19,20,21]

There is great variation in the PRP preparation and application methods used to treat AGA patients.[22,23,24,25,26] This fact may account for some of the variability in response seen in published observational and randomized clinical trials. A recent metaanalysis reported that PRP was successful in treating patients with AGA, using hair density as the measure of treatment success, as compared to baseline measurements across direct injection studies with an overall standardized mean difference of 0.51 (95% confidence interval: 0.14, 0.88, $I^2 = 0\%$, 4 studies).[26] Additionally, in uncontrolled studies, improvements in hair count, hair density, hair thickness, and microscopic evaluations are frequently reported in AGA patients treated with PRP.[22,24,25,27,28,29,30] Erythema, edema, headaches, drowsiness, mild pain, temporary swelling, and scalp sensitivity were among the common side effects reported.[26] The majority of PRP studies conducted in AGA patients are short term, with only a few studies evaluating past 6 months, thus long-term benefits are hard to determine.[24,25,30]

The highest level of evidence among PRP AGA studies has been provided by Lee et al, who conducted a randomized clinical trial comparing CD34 + cell-containing, leukocyte-rich PRP (PRP + PDRN) to polydeoxyribonucleotide (PDRN) in female pattern hair loss patients ($n = 40$).[31] PDRN was used in comparison as it can enhance angiogenesis, stimulate wound healing and promote cell regeneration.[32] Twenty patients were treated with 12 weekly sessions of intra-perifollicular PDRN injections, while 20 patients in the active treatment group received 1 session of PRP, followed by 12 weekly sessions of intraperifollicular PDRN injections. Greater improvement in hair thickness occurred in the PRP + PDRN treatment group as compared to the PDRN comparator ($p = 0.031$).[31] One week after their final session, improvements in hair counts and hair thickness were noted in both treatment groups as compared to baseline measurements.[31] Evidence of PRP's success has also been found in recent clinical trials conducted in AGA patients, supporting the use of PRP as a treatment for AGA.[33,34,35]

4.3 PRP for Alopecia Areata

Alopecia areata (AA, also referred to as spot or patch baldness) is an autoimmune hair loss condition where the immune system attacks actively growing hair follicles.[36] This condition commonly occurs on the scalp but may involve other facial or body hairs and affects both men and women.[37,38] There are currently no FDA approved therapies for AA; however, many off-label medications (e.g., intralesional triamcinolone, minoxidil) have shown some efficacy. The anti-inflammatory effects of PRP may be of value to these patients. Importantly, studies regarding the management of AA should be interpreted cautiously, since the disease has an unpredictable natural history with spontaneous remissions and relapses.

Intralesional triamcinolone acetonide injections are first-line treatment in many cases of AA. However, a single placebo- and active-controlled, double-blinded, split-scalp, randomized clinical trial found that PRP may be a more efficacious treatment option. Trink et al injected half the scalp in 45 patients with PRP, triamcinolone acetonide, or placebo monthly for

3 months and found a higher success rate, defined as complete remission, among PRP treated lesions (60%) as compared to the steroid (27%).[39] PRP also provided greater success in regrowing fully pigmented hair, with 96% of PRP-treated AA patients regrowing pigmented hairs as compared to 25% of triamcinolone acetonide-treated AA patients.[39] Regrowth in PRP-treated patients has also been reported to occur earlier than minoxidil-treated patients as determined in a placebo-controlled study.[40] This earlier response may not occur in all AA types as PRP is not effective against alopecia totalis.[40] Case reports also suggest that PRP can be a promising treatment for AA.[41]

Taken together, there is some evidence that PRP may be beneficial in treating AA. However, studies are few, some lack control, and generally are small in size. The authors have had limited success treating AA with PRP and believe that alternative therapies such as JAK kinases inhibitors are more.

4.4 PRP for Cicatricial Alopecia

Cicatricial alopecia (scarring alopecia) is a rarer class of hair loss comprised of several different and often overlapping conditions such as central centrifugal cicatrical alopecia (CCCA), lichen planopilaris (LPP), frontal fibrosing alopecia (FFA), traction alopecia, etc. All of these diseases result in folliscular damage and eventually permanent replacement with fibrous tissue.[42] Histopathological diagnosis and management of scarring alopecia can be challenging with the primary goal of minimizing inflammation and preserving existing hairs. Restoration options, such as hair transplantation and tissue expansion techniques, can be limited and are only considered after scarring has become fixed.[43,44,45]

Theoretically, PRP may be of value in these hair loss patients, as it has both regenerative and anti-inflammatory properties.

Evidence supporting the use of PRP in scarring alopecia is limited. There are no large-scale randomized controlled trials, but case studies suggest that PRP may be beneficial in some types of CA.[43] Several months after the combination of a hair transplantation and PRP treatment, an LPP patient was able to achieve a high graft survival rate (approximately 80%), suggesting PRP may be advantageous following surgical hair restoration procedures.[43]

While PRP could be beneficial, in the authors' experience, success is limited for both AA and CA. They believe the future lies in treatment of both conditions with JAK kinase inhibitors (orally and topically) rather than PRP.

4.5 PRP with Surgical Hair Restoration

Follicular unit transplantation (FUT) and follicular unit extraction (FUE) are the main hair transplant options available to AGA patients. During FUT, hair follicles are obtained through the surgical removal of a hair-bearing strip from the back of the scalp. As an alternative to FUT, follicular units can be harvested individually from the donor region using the FUE harvesting technique. During both FUE and FUT, hair follicles are subject to injury or dehydration[46] and thus, less viable. Graft storage solutions containing activated platelets could help with graft preservation and encourage grafts to enter the anagen (growth) phase prior to implantation (▶ Fig. 4.2).[10,47] When grafts were soaked in PRP solution prior to FUT, a 15% increase in hair growth and hair density was reported as compared to grafts soaked in saline solution.[47] PRP can also be used successfully in FUE

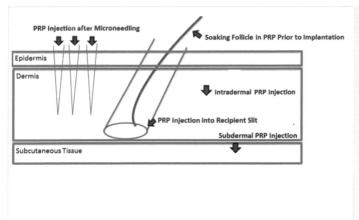

Fig. 4.2 Possible locations to inject PRP. (Adapted from Puig CJ, Reese R, Peters M. Double-Blind, Placebo-Controlled Pilot Study on the Use of Platelet-Rich Plasma in Women With Female Androgenetic Alopecia. Dermatol Surg Off Publ Am Soc Dermatol Surg Al. 2016 Nov;42(11):1243–7, Garg S. Outcome of Intra-operative Injected Platelet-rich Plasma Therapy During Follicular Unit Extraction Hair Transplant: A Prospective Randomised Study in Forty Patients. J Cutan Aesthetic Surg. 2016 Sep;9(3):157–64, and Rogers N. Review of the Literature: Microneedling for Hair Loss? Hair Transpl Forum Int. 2016;26(1):39.)

procedures as evident in a single-blind, randomized study of 40 patients with AGA.[48] In this study, a greater number of PRP treated patients had increased hair regrowth and hair density after FUE as compared to non-PRP treated patients (20/20 = 100% vs. 4/20 = 20% and 12/20 = 60% vs. 0/20 = 0%, respectively).[48]

4.5.1 Important Techniques to Consider

There are a number of important techniques that may be of value when creating a PRP protocol, such as exogenous versus autoactivation. Additional of thrombin and calcium chloride to the solution can activate platelets and trigger degranulation of α-granules.[7,49,50] This degranulation can enhance the release of specific growth factors such as insulin-like growth factor 1 (IGF-1) and PDGF.[7,49,50] However, activation may not always lead to better hair restoration results.[35] Additionally, activation may not necessarily result in better hair restoration outcomes as significant change in the concentration of some growth factors does not always occur.[24,25,27,28,35] Thus, further research into identifying which

activated growth factors and collection systems can achieve the best hair restoration outcomes is needed. Head-to-head clinical trials will help optimize treatment protocols and inform clinicians about how to best prepare their PRP solutions.

Extracellular matrix (ECM) materials can also be added to PRP to enhance hair restoration outcomes. ECM materials can encourage stem cells to form progenitor cells that may protect dermal papilla cells against the effects of increased DHT levels (e.g., follicle miniaturization).[51,52] Similar to PRP, ECM materials contain growth factors promoting hair growth such as VEGF, epidermal growth factor (EGF), and insulin like growth factor (IGF).[53,54] Some regulatory bodies (e.g., FDA) have approved the use of porcine derived urinary bladder ECM material (ACell MatriStem, ACell Inc., Columbia, MD) to help repair and remodel damaged tissues.[55,56] ECM materials in combination with PRP can be used to improve wound healing and donor scarring during surgical hair restoration procedures.[57,58,59] But, products such as Acell contain foreign proteins, so the possibility of a reaction to this material increases the potential for side effects over PRP alone.

Furthermore, the increased extracellular pressure of injecting a dense material near follicles could possibly cause negative responses. Without good studies to document improvement with ECM materials and to quantify these risks, it is difficult to substantiate its use. Further research with randomized controlled clinical trials is required as few studies have explored these combined regenerative therapies in alopecia patients.

Single- and double-spin methods can be used to create PRP solutions.[25,60] The first spin can allow the red blood cells to separate from the plasma.[60] Avoiding high speeds and long durations are encouraged as platelets can be precipitated.[60] Additionally, high concentrations of red or white blood cells in PRP solutions can cause inflammation adjacent to the follicle and be deleterious to hair growth; thus, it is best to limit the amount of red and white blood cells in the final injected preparation.[61] Platelets

can be further separated in a second spin. During this second spin, the goal is to precipitate platelets; therefore, higher speeds and longer durations may be helpful. Caution is still advised, however, as high speeds may discharge PDGF from platelets and limit its eventual deposition in the scalp.[60] Both single- and double-spin methods can achieve high volume PRP yields and create desired hair restoration results.[33,48,62] Fully automated collection systems, such as the Magellan Autologous Platelet Separator system, can also be used to separate and concentrate platelets.[63]

To achieve optimum results, it is suggested that PRP should be performed once a month for 3 months with a platelet concentration of 4 to 7 times a patient's baseline whole blood levels (▶ Fig. 4.3, ▶ Fig. 4.4, ▶ Fig. 4.5, ▶ Fig. 4.6, ▶ Fig. 4.7, ▶ Fig. 4.8, ▶ Fig. 4.9, ▶ Fig. 4.10, ▶ Fig. 4.11, ▶ Fig. 4.12).[64,65] PRP injections can be administered intradermally, subdermally,

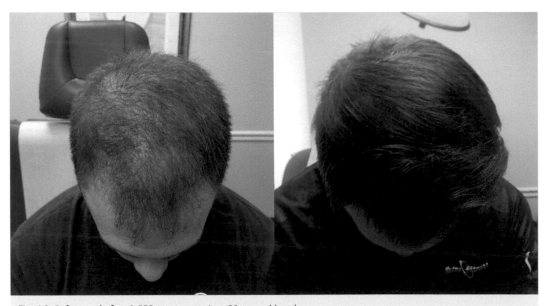

Fig. 4.3 Before and after 9 PRP treatments in a 29-year-old male.

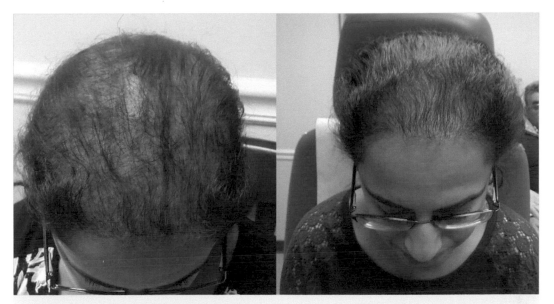

Fig. 4.4 Before and after 6 PRP treatments in a 43-year-old female.

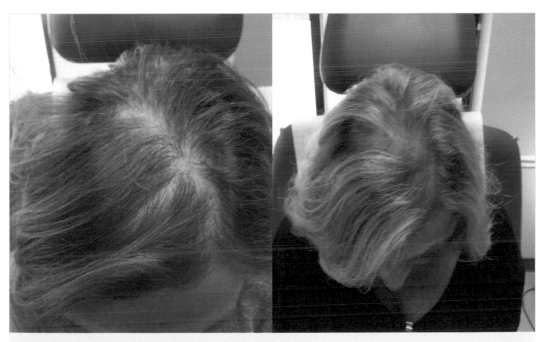

Fig. 4.5 Before and after 5 PRP treatments in a 67-year-old patient.

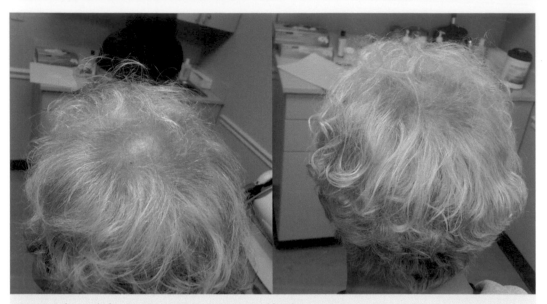

Fig. 4.6 Before and after 3 PRP treatments in a 61-year-old male.

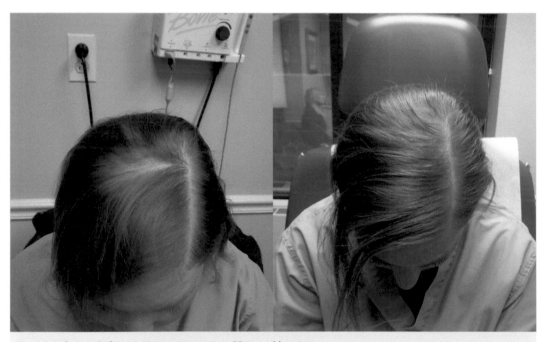

Fig. 4.7 Before and after 13 PRP treatments in a 27-year-old patient.

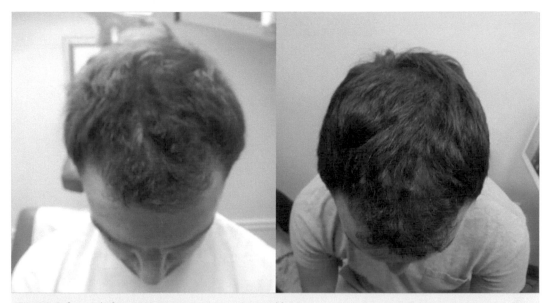

Fig. 4.8 Before and after 4 PRP treatments in an 18-year-old patient.

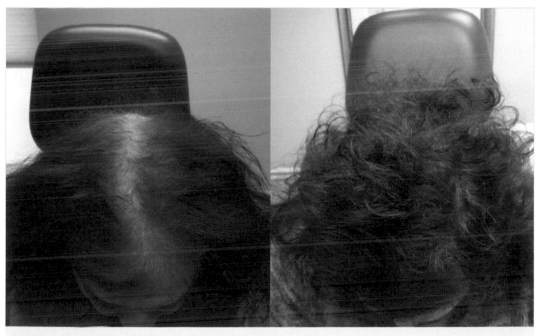

Fig. 4.9 Before and after 11 PRP treatments in a 61-year-old patient.

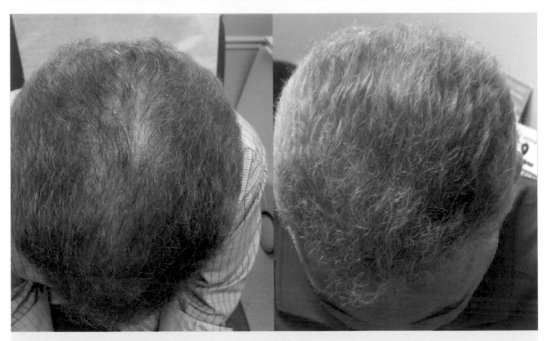

Fig. 4.10 Before and after 7 PRP treatments in a 47-year-old male patient.

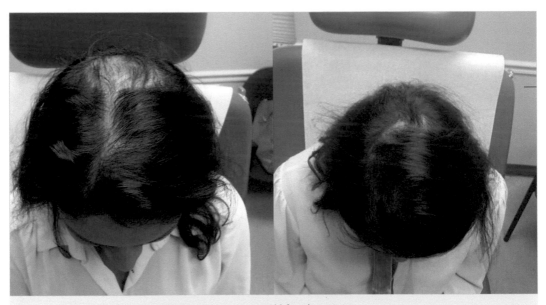

Fig. 4.11 Before and after 7 PRP treatments in a 47-year-old female patient.

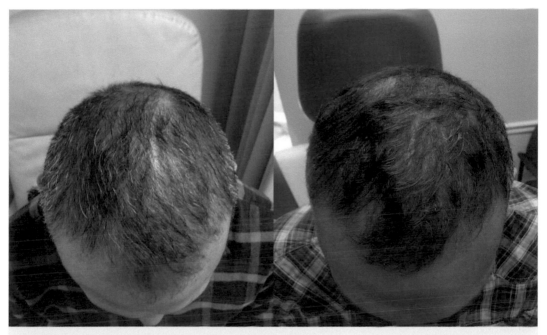

Fig. 4.12 Before and after 7 PRP treatments in a 54-year-old patient.

and/or placed into premade recipient slits and microneedling channels (▶ Fig. 4.2).[34, 48,66] It is the authors' opinion that subdermal injections (e.g., Rapaport Subdermal Depo PRP injection) are preferred over intradermal injections, so direct delivery of PRP to the base of the hair follicle can occur. Subdermal injections can also allow for better diffusion of PRP in the loose connective tissue space, effectively coating the hair follicle and decreasing the number of injections necessary to bathe a given area.[67] This technique is well tolerated and may be less painful because as the solution diffuses there is less local pressure than when it exerts pressure on the dermis. These recommendations are only guidelines as standardized PRP procedures have yet to be determined and no studies directly compare one injection technique to the other.

4.6 Conclusion

To conclude, PRP therapy is a promising noninvasive hair restoration option, since PRP encourages hair growth, cell survival, and angiogenesis. Short-term studies suggest that PRP produces positive results, including increased hair density and improved hair restoration outcomes with better graft survival and less scar formation, among patients with AGA. There is also some evidence among patients suffering from AA. As only case studies have been conducted in management of CA, more research is required to determine how applicable PRP therapy is to scarring alopecia. Randomized clinical trials should seek to standardize and optimize PRP techniques for the treatment of alopecia, as this could help achieve consistent results and allow for better patient counseling.

References

[1] Spindler JR. The safety of topical minoxidil solution in the treatment of pattern baldness: the results of a 27-center trial. Clin Dermatol. 1988; 6(4):200–212

[2] PROPECIA (finasteride) tablets for oral use. U.S. Food and Drug Administration. 2014 Available at: http://www.accessdata.fda.gov/drugsatfda_docs/label/2014/020788s024lbl.pdf. Accessed June 8, 2017

[3] Monograph P. Hair Regrowth Forumula. Minoxidil Topical Solution USP 20 mg/mL (2% w/v). Health Canada. Drug Product Database. 2016. Available at: https://health-products.canada.ca/dpd-bdpp/dispatch-repartition.do. Accessed June 6, 2017

[4] Men's Rogaine. 5% Minoxidil Topical Aerosol. Hair Regrowth Treatment. U.S. Food and Drug Administration. 2015. Available at: http://www.accessdata.fda.gov/drugsatfda_docs/label/2006/021812s000LBL.pdf. Accessed October 6, 2016

[5] Gupta AK, Carviel J, MacLeod MA, Shear N. Assessing finasteride-associated sexual dysfunction using the FAERS database. J Eur Acad Dermatol Venereol. 2017; 31(6):1069–1075

[6] Knudsen RG. The challenge of FUE in women. Hair Transpl Forum International.. 2014; 24(4):150

[7] Gupta AK, Carviel J. A mechanistic model of platelet-rich plasma treatment for androgenetic alopecia. Dermatol Surg. 2016; 42(12):1335–1339

[8] Okuda K, Kawase T, Momose M, et al. Platelet-rich plasma contains high levels of platelet-derived growth factor and transforming growth factor-beta and modulates the proliferation of periodontally related cells in vitro. J Periodontol. 2003; 74(6):849–857

[9] Eppley BL, Woodell JE, Higgins J. Platelet quantification and growth factor analysis from platelet-rich plasma: implications for wound healing. Plast Reconstr Surg. 2004; 114(6):1502–1508

[10] Li ZJ, Choi H-I, Choi D-K, et al. Autologous platelet-rich plasma: a potential therapeutic tool for promoting hair growth. Dermatol Surg. 2012; 38(7 Pt 1):1040–1046

[11] El-Sharkawy H, Kantarci A, Deady J, et al. Platelet-rich plasma: growth factors and pro- and anti-inflammatory properties. J Periodontol. 2007; 78(4):661–669

[12] Shumez H, Prasad P, Kaviarasan P, Deepika R. Intralesional platelet rich plasma vs intralesional triamcinolone in the treatment of alopecia areata: a comparative study. Int J Med Res Health Sci. 2014; 4(1):118–122

[13] Gilhar A, Etzioni A, Paus R. Alopecia areata. N Engl J Med. 2012; 366(16):1515–1525

[14] Hudgens JL, Sugg KB, Grekin JA, Gumucio JP, Bedi A, Mendias CL. Platelet-rich plasma activates proinflammatory signaling pathways and induces oxidative stress in tendon fibroblasts. Am J Sports Med. 2016; 44(8):1931–1940

[15] Schweikert HU, Wilson JD. Regulation of human hair growth by steroid hormones. II. Androstenedione metabolism in isolated hairs. J Clin Endocrinol Metab. 1974; 39(6):1012–1019

[16] Sawaya ME, Price VH. Different levels of 5alpha-reductase type I and II, aromatase, and androgen receptor in hair follicles of women and men with androgenetic alopecia. J Invest Dermatol. 1997; 109(3):296–300

[17] Levy-Nissenbaum E, Bar-Natan M, Frydman M, Pras E. Confirmation of the association between male pattern baldness and the androgen receptor gene. Eur J Dermatol. 2005; 15(5):339–340

[18] Semalty M, Semalty A, Joshi GP, Rawat MSM. Hair growth and rejuvenation: an overview. J Dermatolog Treat. 2011; 22 (3):123–132

[19] Lattanand A, Johnson WC. Male pattern alopecia a histopathologic and histochemical study. J Cutan Pathol. 1975; 2(2):58–70

[20] Abell E. Histologic response to topically applied minoxidil in male-pattern alopecia. Clin Dermatol. 1988; 6(4):191–194

[21] Whiting D. Inflammation and hair loss. 20th World Congress of Dermatology, Paris; July 2002

[22] Takikawa M, Nakamura S, Nakamura S, et al. Enhanced effect of platelet-rich plasma containing a new carrier on hair growth. Dermatol Surg. 2011; 37(12):1721–1729

[23] Borhan R, Gasnier C, Reygagne P. Autologous platelet rich plasma as a treatment of male androgenetic alopecia: study of 14 cases. Journal of Clinical and Experimental Dermatology Research 2015;06(04). Available at: http://www.omicsonline.org/open-access/autologous-platelet-rich-plasma-as-a-treatment-of-male-androgenetic-alopecia-study-of-14-cases-2155-9554-10000292.php?aid=57866. Accessed June 26, 2017

[24] Cervelli V, Garcovich S, Bielli A, et al. The effect of autologous activated platelet rich plasma (AA-PRP) injection on pattern hair loss: clinical and histomorphometric evaluation. BioMed Res Int. 2014; 2014:760709

[25] Gkini M-A, Kouskoukis A-E, Tripsianis G, Rigopoulos D, Kouskoukis K. Study of platelet-rich plasma injections in the treatment of androgenetic alopecia through an one-year period. J Cutan Aesthet Surg. 2014; 7(4):213–219

[26] Gupta AK, Carviel JL. Meta-analysis of efficacy of platelet-rich plasma therapy for androgenetic alopecia. J Dermatolog Treat. 2017; 28(1):55–58

[27] Singhal P, Agarwal S, Dhot PS, Sayal SK. Efficacy of platelet-rich plasma in treatment of androgenic alopecia. Asian J Transfus Sci. 2015; 9(2):159–162

[28] Khatu SS, More YE, Gokhale NR, Chavhan DC, Bendsure N. Platelet-rich plasma in androgenic alopecia: myth or an effective tool. J Cutan Aesthet Surg. 2014; 7(2):107–110

[29] Betsi EE, Germain E, Kalbermatten DF, Tremp M, Emmenegger V. Platelet-rich plasma injection is effective and safe for the treatment of alopecia. Eur J Plast Surg. 2013; 36(7):407–412

[30] Gentile P, Garcovich S, Bielli A, Scioli MG, Orlandi A, Cervelli V. The effect of platelet-rich plasma in hair regrowth: a randomized placebo-controlled trial. Stem Cells Transl Med. 2015; 4(11):1317–1323

[31] Lee S-H, Zheng Z, Kang J-S, Kim D-Y, Oh SH, Cho SB. Therapeutic efficacy of autologous platelet-rich plasma and polydeoxyribonucleotide on female pattern hair loss. Wound Repair Regen. 2015; 23(1):30–36

[32] Yu M, Lee JY. Polydeoxyribonucleotide improves wound healing of fractional laser resurfacing in rat model. J Cosmet Laser Ther. 2017; 19(1):43–48

[33] Gupta S, Revathi TN, Sacchidanand S, Nataraj HV. A study of the efficacy of platelet-rich plasma in the treatment of androgenetic alopecia in males. Indian J Dermatol Venereol Leprol. 2017; 83(3):412

[34] Puig CJ, Reese R, Peters M. Double-blind, placebo-controlled pilot study on the use of platelet-rich plasma in women with female androgenetic alopecia. Dermatol Surg. 2016; 42(11):1243–1247

[35] Gentile P, Cole JP, Cole MA, et al. Evaluation of not-activated and activated prp in hair loss treatment: role of growth factor and cytokine concentrations obtained by different collection systems. Int J Mol Sci. 2017; 18(2):E408

[36] McMichael AJ, Pearce DJ, Wasserman D, et al. Alopecia in the United States: outpatient utilization and common prescribing patterns. J Am Acad Dermatol. 2007; 57(2) Suppl:S49–S51

[37] Finner AM. Alopecia areata: clinical presentation, diagnosis, and unusual cases. Dermatol Ther (Heidelb). 2011; 24(3): 348–354

[38] Alkhalifah A, Alsantali A, Wang E, McElwee KJ, Shapiro J. Alopecia areata update: part I. Clinical picture, histopathology, and pathogenesis. J Am Acad Dermatol. 2010; 62(2):177–188, quiz 189–190

[39] Trink A, Sorbellini E, Bezzola P, et al. A randomized, double-blind, placebo- and active-controlled, half-head study to evaluate the effects of platelet-rich plasma on alopecia areata. Br J Dermatol. 2013; 169(3):690–694

[40] El Taieb MA, Ibrahim H, Nada EA, Seif Al-Din M. Platelets rich plasma versus minoxidil 5% in treatment of alopecia areata: A trichoscopic evaluation. Dermatol Ther (Heidelb). 2017; 30(1):1–6

[41] Donovan J. Successful treatment of corticosteroid-resistant ophiasis-type alopecia areata (AA) with platelet-rich plasma (PRP). JAAD Case Rep. 2015; 1(5):305–307

[42] Harries MJ, Sinclair RD, Macdonald-Hull S, Whiting DA, Griffiths CEM, Paus R. Management of primary cicatricial alopecias: options for treatment. Br J Dermatol. 2008; 159(1):1–22

[43] Saxena K, Saxena DK, Savant SS. Successful hair transplant outcome in cicatricial lichen planus of the scalp by combining scalp and beard hair along with platelet rich plasma. J Cutan Aesthet Surg. 2016; 9(1):51–55

[44] Unger W, Unger R, Wesley C. The surgical treatment of cicatricial alopecia. Dermatol Ther (Heidelb). 2008; 21(4): 295–311

[45] Fan J-C, Wang J-P. Plastic surgical management of large cicatricial scalp alopecia. Zhonghua Yi Xue Za Zhi. 2009; 89(16): 1098–1101

[46] Zontos G, Rose PT, Nikiforidis G. A mathematical proof of how the outgrowth angle of hair follicles influences the injury to the donor area in FUE harvesting. Dermatol Surg. 2014; 40(10):1147–1150

[47] Uebel CO, da Silva JB, Cantarelli D, Martins P. The role of platelet plasma growth factors in male pattern baldness surgery. Plast Reconstr Surg. 2006; 118(6):1458–1466, discussion 1467

[48] Garg S. Outcome of intra-operative injected platelet-rich plasma therapy during follicular unit extraction hair transplant: a prospective randomised study in forty patients. J Cutan Aesthet Surg. 2016; 9(3):157–164

[49] Arshdeep, Kumaran MS. Platelet-rich plasma in dermatology: boon or a bane? Indian J Dermatol Venereol Leprol. 2014; 80 (1):5–14

[50] Vogt PM, Lehnhardt M, Wagner D, Jansen V, Krieg M, Steinau HU. Determination of endogenous growth factors in human wound fluid: temporal presence and profiles of secretion. Plast Reconstr Surg. 1998; 102(1):117–123

[51] Hitzig G. Regenerative medicine part 1: usage of porcine extracellular matrix in hair loss prevention, hair restoration surgery and donor scar revision. In: Lam S, ed. Hair Transplant 360. New Delhi, India: Jaypee Brothers Publishing; 2014:553–564

[52] Beattie AJ, Gilbert TW, Guyot JP, Yates AJ, Badylak SF. Chemoattraction of progenitor cells by remodeling extracellular matrix scaffolds. Tissue Eng Part A. 2009; 15(5):1119–1125

[53] Badylak SF. The extracellular matrix as a scaffold for tissue reconstruction. Semin Cell Dev Biol. 2002; 13(5):377–383

[54] Badylak SF. Xenogeneic extracellular matrix as a scaffold for tissue reconstruction. Transpl Immunol. 2004; 12(3–4):367–377

[55] ACELL, Inc. Receives new FDA clearances, prepares for future growth. ACell. 2015. Available at: https://acell.com/acell-inc-receives-new-fda-clearances-prepares-for-future-growth/. Accessed July 24, 2017

[56] ACELL, Inc. Receives FDA clearance for concurrent use of its wound management devices. ACell. 2016. Available at: https://acell.com/acell-inc-receives-fda-clearance-for-concurrent-use-of-its-wound-management-devices/. [July 24, 2017

[57] Cooley J.. Use of porcine bladder matrix in hair restoration surgery applications. Hair Transpl Forum Int. 2011; 21(3):65, 71–72

[58] Puig C. Use of PRP and dermal matrix. Presented at: Annual Meeting of the American Academy of Cosmetic Surgery; January 14; 2015; New Orleans, LA. Lecture

[59] Rose PT. Hair restoration surgery: challenges and solutions. Clin Cosmet Investig Dermatol. 2015; 8:361–370

[60] Fukaya M, Ito A. A New Economic Method for Preparing Platelet-rich Plasma. Plast Reconstr Surg Glob Open. 2014; 2(6):e162

[61] Wu Y, Kanna MS, Liu C, Zhou Y, Chan CK. Generation of autologous platelet-rich plasma by the ultrasonic standing waves. IEEE Trans Biomed Eng. 2016; 63(8):1642–1652

[62] About Eclipse PRP. Eclipse. Available at: http://eclipseaesthetics.com/products/eclipse-prp/. Accessed August 7, 2017

[63] Arthrex Research and Development. Angel vs Magellan: A Comparative Study on Platelet Concentration and Activation. 2015. Available at: https://www.arthrex.com/resources/white-paper/pS5iTVoznkqc0QFQPdjYQQ/angel-vs-magellan-a-comparative-study-on-platelet-concentration-and-activation. Accessed August 7, 2017

[64] Godse K. Platelet-rich plasma in androgenic alopecia: where do we stand? J Cutan Aesthet Surg. 2014; 7(2):110–111

[65] Marx RE. Platelet-rich plasma (PRP): what is PRP and what is not PRP? Implant Dent. 2001; 10(4):225–228

[66] Rogers N. Review of the literature: microneedling for hair loss? Hair Transpl Forum Int. 2016; 26(1):39

[67] Bellomo R, Rapaport J. Incorporating platelet-rich plasma for hair restoration into your practice. The Dermatologist. 2017; 25(3). Available at https://www.the-dermatologist.com/content/incorporating-platelet-rich-plasma-hair-restoration-your-practice. Accessed February 12, 2019

Part II

Microneedling Principles and Practices

II

5
Microneedling: Mechanism and Practical Considerations

Amelia K. Hausauer

Abstract

Microneedling has become an increasingly popular procedure to treat a variety of cutaneous conditions. It involves disruption of the epidermis and/or dermis by fine-gauged needles attached to a stamp, roller, or mechanized pen. Although a detailed mechanism of action remains unclear, there are two competing hypotheses: fractionated mechanical injury triggering wound healing cascades, and demarcation current—intercellular electrical shifts—stimulating signaling molecules and deoxyribonucleic acid (DNA) synthesis. Irrespective of the exact molecular pathways, histologic studies suggest that microneedling leads to epidermal thickening, collagen induction, elastic fiber proliferation, and neoangiogeneis. Understanding difference in delivery systems and appropriate clinical parameters is critical to achieve these desired tissue changes.

Keywords: microneedling, collagen induction therapy, mechanism of action, fractionated mechanical injury, demarcation current, wound healing, growth factors, technical considerations, clinical considerations

Key Points

- Microneedling has evolved over recent decades and has multiple uses in dermatology.

- Complete understanding of microneedling's mechanism of action is unknown. There are two leading hypotheses: (1) fractionated mechanical microinjury with classical wound healing and (2) demarcation current during which shifts in transepithelial electrical potential leads to cellular migration, proliferation, and remodeling. Stimulation of growth factors and DNA synthesis pathways plays a crucial role in the downstream effects.
- There are three main device types: stamps, rollers, and pens. Each has advantages and disadvantages. Needles vary as well.
- Providers should understand which systems to use in different clinician scenarios and how to tailor treatments to anatomic location and cutaneous condition.

5.1 Introduction

An increasingly popular, minimally invasive procedure, microneedling combines the ancient principles of acupuncture and mesotherapy with more modern technologies to treat a range of cutaneous conditions. In the 1990s, Orentreich and Orentreich first reported "subcision" involving the use of a needle inserted parallel to the skin's surface to manually disrupt scars, a procedure best suited for small treatment areas given the risk of bruising.[1] Camirand and Doucet then treated scars using a tattoo gun to break dermally tethered collagen bands, but this technique was labor intensive and slow with little control over the depth of penetration.[2] Fernandes subsequently built upon these principles in his seminal paper from 2005 and coined the term "percutaneous collagen induction" (PCI) therapy, referring to rejuvenation and skin remodeling with tiny needles mounted on a cylindrical roller (also known as derma-roller).[3] Since this time, the technique has undergone several iterations with its avatars including collagen induction therapy, dermal needling, dry tattooing, intradermabrasion, and microneedling.

5.2 Mechanism(s) of Action

Microneedling involves the production of transient epidermal and dermal pores ranging from 25 to 3,000 μm in depth with the fundamental goal of upregulating normal skin synthesis mechanisms

and not inducing prolonged inflammation or trauma that may lead to fibrosis. There are two major theories explaining how needles induce tissue remodeling and proliferation.

5.2.1 Fractionated Mechanical Microinjury

The first explanation involves what the authors like to refer to as *fractionated mechanical microinjury* (▶ Fig. 5.1). Needling forms tightly packed, minute perforations. The resultant near-confluent dermal and superficial capillary disruption provides a strong stimulus for growth factor release and fibroblast infiltration.[4,5,6,7]

Microchannels heal following the three classic phases of wound healing: inflammatory, proliferation, and remodeling. In reality, these phases overlap and a full discussion of the process is beyond the scope of this chapter. However, briefly, the inflammatory phase begins when disruption of the stratum corneum, endothelial lining, and subendothelial

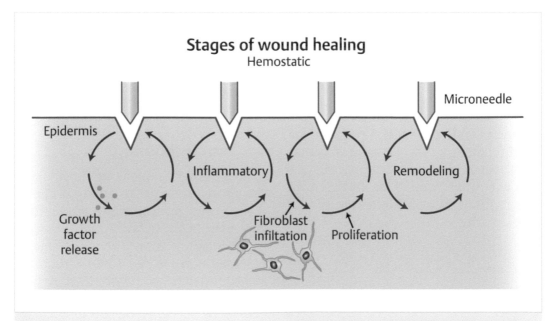

Fig. 5.1 Fractional mechanical microinjury hypothesis for the mechanism of action in microneedling. Tiny, superficial wounds form a strong stimulus for growth factor release and fibroblast infiltration following the classical phases of healing.

matrix recruits platelets and neutrophils to the site of injury. Needling expose thrombin and collagen fragments, which attract and activate platelets locally within minutes. The platelets, in turn, form a plug, initiate clotting, and release a myriad of growth factors and cytokines (▶ Table 5.1). These signaling molecules control clot formation, increase vascular permeability, and attract leukocytes and fibroblasts to the site of injury. In the first 48 hours, neutrophils predominate; however, it is the subsequent influx of macrophages that is critical not only for phagocytosis but also to perpetuate signaling cascades that induces cell migration and division—without which healing fails to occur.[3,7]

Table 5.1 Important growth factors, cytokines, and other signaling molecules necessary for wound healing and cutaneous remodeling

Molecule	Abbre-viation	Functions
Fibroblast growth factor	FGF	• Fibroblast, epithelial cell proliferation • Matrix deposition • Angiogenesis • wound contract
Platelet-derived growth factor	PDGF	• Fibroblast, macrophage, neutrophil chemotaxis • Fibroblast, epithelial, smooth muscle cell, mesanchymal cell proliferation • Collagen metabolism • Angiogenesis
Transforming growth factor alpha	TGF-α	• Keratinocyte migration, proliferation (reepithelialization)
Transforming growth factor beta	TGF-β	• Fibroblast chemotaxis, proliferation • Collagen, matrix metabolism • Protease inhibition • Angiogenesis • Immunomodulation TGF-β1 and TGF-β2 are profibrotic while TGF-β3 is antifibrotic
Epidermal growth factor	EGF	• Keratinocyte migration, proliferation

Table 5.1 continued

Molecule	Abbre-viation	Functions
		• Fibroblast, endothelial cell, mesenchymal cell proliferation and modulation • Angiogenesis • Collagenase regulation
Insulin-like growth factor 1	IGF-1	• Keratinocyte migration, proliferation • Fibroblast chemotaxis • Protein synthesis
Vascular endothelial growth factor	VEGF	• Angiogenesis • Vascular permeability • Endothelial cell chemotaxis, proliferation • Macrophage chemotaxis
Connective tissue growth factor	CTGF	• Fibroblast chemotaxis, proliferation • Collagen metabolism • Angiogenesis • Platelet adhesion • Fibrosis
Keratinocyte growth factor	KGF	• Keratinocyte proliferation
Connective tissue activating peptide III		• Matrix proliferation, production
Neutrophil activating peptide-2		• Neutrophil chemotaxis
Interleukin 1	IL-1	• Fibroblast proliferation • Collagenase regulation-3 (MMP-13) • Pro-inflammation, pyrogen
Interleukin 10	IL-10	• Collagen remodeling • MMP gene expression • Anti-inflammation

Abbreviation: MMP, matrix metalloproteinases.
Note: This table is intended as an overview and is not exhaustive.[3,8,9,10,11]

This also marks a transition to the proliferative phase of wound healing, during which growth factors derived from macrophages (i.e., PDGF [platelet-derived growth factor], TGF-α [transforming growth factor] and TGF-β, interleukin-1, tumor necrosis factor, FGF [fibroblast growth factor]) recruit fibroblasts and alter extracellular matrix synthesis. Fibroblasts migrating along a fibronectin scaffold allow for fibroplasia and granulation of the wound. Typically in healing of larger wounds, keratinocytes change their phenotype and migrate to repair tears in the basement membrane. Desmosomes dissolve and actin forms to knit keratinocytes together. The small injuries created by microneedles disrupt the basement membrane and expose keratinocytes to dermal collagen, thereby stimulating multiplication. However, these defects are miniscule and close rapidly—within hours—so the proliferating keratinocytes serve more to thicken the epidermis rather than close the needling channels.[3,7,12]

At the same time, relative tissue hypoxia is another cue that triggers cytokine release, in response to which fibroblasts produce PDGF, FGF, and EGF. There is an upregulation of procollagen mRNA, which later converts to collagen III in the presence of oxygen supplied by new vessels.[3,6] VEGF and other growth factors are key in the angiogenesis process.[6]

The remodeling begins in days with the formation of the fibronectin matrix but takes months to years for full execution. Hence, much of the improvement in skin quality seen after microneedling appears after three to four weeks and continues for months.[13] Collagen type I replaces III, which replaces the early granulation tissue laid down in the upper dermis. Interestingly, this collagen integrates a regular basket-weave lattice rather than in the parallel bundles seen in scars.[13,14,15,16] Assays from needled skin in rats suggest that disproportionately high levels of TGF-β3, an antifibrotic cytokine, may account for the scarless healing seen with microneedling.[8] Vitamin A or retinoic acid favors the production of TGF-β3 over its profibrotic family members TGF-β1 and TGF-β2 and explains why some providers combine topical retinyl esters in their protocol.[8] Some investigators assert that matrix metalloproteinases may also play a crucial role in decreasing the fibrosis and perhaps minimizing hyperpigmentation,[13] yet these mechanisms have not been elucidated fully.

5.2.2 Demarcation Current

Leibl proposed an alternative explanation for the cutaneous effects status post microneedling—shifts in transepithelial potentials called "demarcation current" (▶ Fig. 5.2).'[13] In the resting state, the intracellular potential of epidermal cells is negative (approximately −70 mV), while the extracellular potential is positive. Injury releases intracellular potassium and proteins into the extracellular compartment, further decreasing the negative potential of the intracellular compartment to as low as −120 mV, thereby increasing the potential difference between the interior and exterior of the cell. When this process occurs repeatedly in close proximity, the generated bioelectrical current triggers growth factor cascades that elicit the migration of fibroblasts, which proliferate and produce collagen.[13,17] While deep skin cuts heal via the classic wound healing mechanisms briefly outlined above, superficial injuries produce only minor inflammation and are more likely to interfere with the intracellular electric fields to alter DNA expression and enhance cell motility. Ultimately, the hemostatic, inflammatory, proliferative, and remodeling phases of wound healing are circumvented or curtailed, so repair occurs sans scar formation.[13] This hypothesis may explain why some studies find better results with repeat superficial treatments (1 mm depth) compared to deeper, aggressive needling (3 mm), although that has been explored fully.[8]

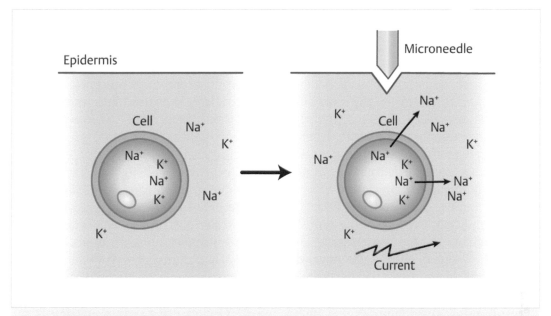

Fig. 5.2 Demarcation current hypothesis for the mechanism of action in microneedling. En masse changes in cell membrane potential create bioelectrical current that changes DNA synthesis and growth factor production. (Adapted from Liebl H and Kloth LC. Skin cell proliferation stimulated by microneedles. J Am Coll Clin Wound Spec 2012;4:2-6.)

5.2.3 Enhanced Drug Delivery

Microneedling enhanced drug delivery to the deeper epidermis and dermis by bypassing the stratum corneum. While often beneficial for increasing the effects of topical medications and cosmeceuticals, the authors urge caution as the risk of adverse inflammatory or other side effects increases when antigenic preparations intended for external use are intradermally deposited (i.e., vitamin C serums).[18]

5.3 Histologic Changes after Microneedling: Basic Science

Several studies use histologic specimens obtained at 3 and/or 6 months after therapy to document microneedling-induced epidermal and dermal changes. Zeittler et al reported epidermal thickening with increased cells in the granular and plus or minus topical vitamin A (retinyl palmitate oil) and C (ascorbyl tetraisopalmitate oil) in an animal model. Compared to unneedled rats, those treated had a denser lattice of thicker collagen fibers and repetitive treatments produced an even more marked response, as seen by Masson's trichrome staining.[8] Interestingly, quantification of *absolute* collagen I and III quantities favored a single treatment over multiple; however, this finding may have been an artifact of study design, since all animals were analyzed 10 weeks after randomization,[8] meaning that the follow-up time from the last needling session differed so histology captured only early neocollagenesis in the repeat treatment groups.

Evidence exists in human skin as well. Aust et al showed that 4 monthly microneedling sessions triggered up to a 400% increase in collagen and elastin deposition by 6 months. This neocollagenesis occurred in a normal basket weave configuration at a depth of up to 0.6 mm with 1.5 mm length needles. At one year, the investigators also noted a thickened stratum spinosum and normal rete ridge architecture compared to the flattening pattern seen over a cicatrix.[16] El-Domyati and colleagues obtained 3 mm punch biopsies at baseline, 1 and 3 months from 10 Fitzpatrick skin type III to IV patients who received a total of six microneedling (1 mm) sessions every 2 weeks to the periorbital and temporal forehead regions. Histologic and immunohistochemical staining showed a statistically significant increase in epidermal thickness at both 1 and 3 months. But, significant boosts in collagen only occurred by three months, corresponding to the progression and sequence of tissue healing. Of note, the total percent of elastin actually decreased, though the precursor to elastin, tropoelastin, rose. While this finding at first seems unfavorable and contradictory to the 6-month data presented by Aust et al, it is likely that evaluation at three months was too early to capture the conversion of tropoelastin to elastin and that by the 6-month time period, the overall elastin content would be higher. Perhaps the increase in tissue elasticity lags behind the rise in collagen, where solar elastotic fibers seen at baseline are cleared (drop in elastin content at 3 months) and trauma induces the production of new precursor elements that are later processed into more normal appearing elastic fibers (rise in elastin content at 6 months).[14,16]

In addition to epidermal and dermal changes, microneedling has been shown to widen the follicular infundibulum by approximately 47% and remove sebum and scale obstructing follicular ostia.[19] These processes enhance topical medication penetration above and beyond the basic concept of breaching the epidermal.

5.4 Technical Considerations

5.4.1 Devices

Evolving from the early subcision[1] and tattooing[2] devices, microneedling systems generally fall into three classes: stamps, rollers, and electronic or mechanical pens (▸ Fig. 5.3). Each has its

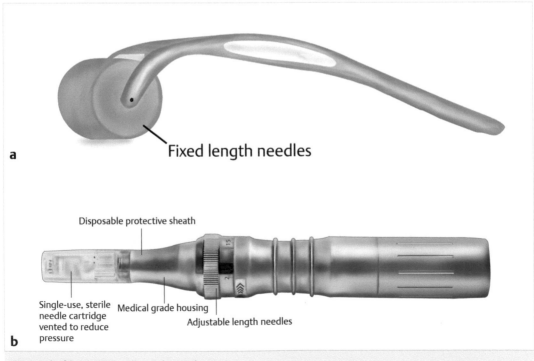

a

Fixed length needles

b

Disposable protective sheath

Single-use, sterile needle cartridge vented to reduce pressure

Medical grade housing

Adjustable length needles

Fig. 5.3 (a, b) Prototype roller and pens devices.

own set of advantages and drawbacks, and many are available only overseas (► Table 5.2).

Table 5.2 Comparison of roller versus electronic devices

Feature	Rollers	Electronic devices
Number of sessions	Single-use (multi if able to clean though no longer sterile) Low possibility of cross contamination	Multiuse hand piece, single-use cartridges Disposable sleeves protects hand piece
Sterility	Most not autoclave safe	Blister-packed, sterile cartridges
Needle depth	Fixed Requires multiple rollers if treatment plan includes different depth	Variable
Device parameters	No need to adjust needle speed or depth Manual pressure and roller rate can be slower down over sensitive areas	Adjustable speed and depth tailored to treatment area or condition Parameters reproducible over multiple sessions
Treatment area	Faster coverage of large areas	Easier access to crevices and contours
Discomfort	More	Less, especially at higher speeds
Cutaneous trauma	Penetrate thicker tissue (i.e., scar) with minimal friction or tearing Curved (not perpendicular) sites of injury, potential risk of tearing skin if improper technique	Require lubrication to glide over skin Many devices have ports to minimize friction Risk of macerating or shearing skin if improper technique
Foreign body reaction	If needle dislodges from cheaper roller	Unlikely
Provider injury	Higher risk for needle stick	Lower risk for needle stick Needles retract when "off"
Cost effectiveness	No initial investment Rollers more expensive	Initial device investment

Table 5.2 continued

Feature	Rollers	Electronic devices
	than cartridges	Cartridges cheaper than rollers

Stamps

Stamps gained popularity in the 1990s but fell out of favor with the advent of rollers. Nevertheless, stamps have several advantages over rollers:

1. They typically cover a small body surface area and can fit more precisely into confined areas such as the upper lip or ala.
2. They do not pull or tangle hair when used on the scalp, especially in longer haired patients.
3. They are usually cost effective for small treatment areas such as scars or for periorificial treatment.[12]

Rollers

Rollers consist of many fine-gauge needles affixed at regular intervals around a drum. Since the needles are set on a cylindrical surface, they enter at an angle, pierce deeper when perpendicular, and exit again at an angle. Hence, the channels created are curved surrounded by intact epidermis with only approximately a four-cell width disruption.[3] It is unclear the clinical relevance of this curved trajectory and whether rolling is more traumatic to the skin than devices that enter orthogonally. Note that vigorous, rapid application of perpendicular needles (stamps, pens) may cause tearing of the epidermis rather than true puncture if performed incorrectly (see below). Dermaroller was the first company to produce a handheld rolling instrument, but now there are many available devices that vary based on needle material, length, caliber, and number (► Table 5.3).

Table 5.3 Needle parameters

Needle material			
	Stainless steel	Most common	
	Titanium	Maintains sharper edge longer	
	Silver, Gold	Antimicrobial, less oxidation, rare risk of allergic reaction	
Needle length			
	0.2–3.0 mm		
Needle diameter			
	Optimal diameter unclear–majority between 30 and 33 gauge		
	>0.25 mm	Potentially higher risk of scarring	
Number of needles			
Rollers	24–1,080	Depends on size and number of rows More rows, shorter treatment time but greater required force and less penetration (Fakir effect)	
Pens	6–18	Device dependent	

Note: Ideal parameters are debated and comparative data is scant.

For any given roller, these parameters are fixed so comprehensive treatment may require more than one device to achieve various depths.

Moreover, it is important to note that cheaper rollers may be flimsy; dull easily; drag along the skin surface, thus creating more collateral damage; and encourage improper grip. Needles may also loosen and dislodge more easily. If they imbed in the skin, foreign body reaction may occur.[3,7,20]

Pens

Developed to overcome some of the limitations associated with rollers, corded or battery-operated pens are the newest technology (► Fig. 5.4). Most utilize sterile, single-use cartridges with needles that oscillate rapidly at either fixed or adjustable frequency. Needle speed helps determine treatment

intensity. Rapid vibration is often less painful, while higher speed, higher power devices bury needles more deeply. Needle length is another adjustable parameter such that a single cartridge can treat multiple body sites at multiple different depths (► Fig. 5.5). Pens are also convenient for crevices and contours, because tips have a small diameter (often 5 mm) relative to bulky roller barrels, and can be either stamped or glided over the skin's surface. As mentioned above, when gliding, it is important that the practitioner's hand move at a rate similar to the needle oscillation so that the needles enter perpendicular. If too rapid, they either skate along the surface without achieving the desire depth or shear the epidermis causing unintended trauma.

Other important features found on some but not all pens include: venting to limit skin drag and fluid build-up; tilting needle plates that adjust to the skin's angle; disposable sterile sleeve to cover the hand piece; and on/off foot pedal.

Needles

There are also several different needle designs, including: solid, coated, dissolving, hallow, and swellable (► Fig. 5.6).[7] Selection depends on the treatment objective. Solid microneedles are the most common. However, hallow needles can effectively deliver vaccines or medications dermally, while coated or insulated needles are often used in radiofrequency devices because the coating protects epidermal melanin from excess heating and limits adverse effects (Chapter 7). ► Table 5.3 outlines several other important features of microneedles.

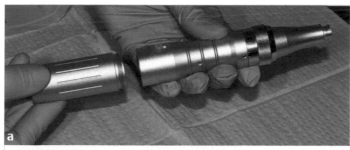
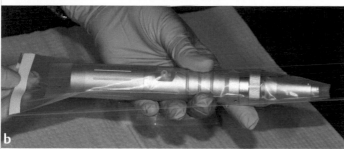
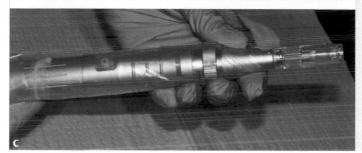

Fig. 5.4 Key components and assembly of a representative microneedling pen for in-office use. **(a)** Attachment of battery followed by **(b)** fitting of proactive sleeve and **(c)** single-use, sterile needle cartridge.

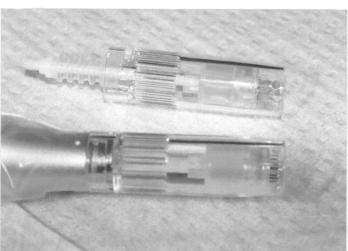

Fig. 5.5 Adjustable needle length 0.25 and 2.0 mm.

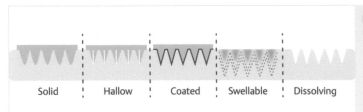

Fig. 5.6 Examples of different types of needles.

Solid | Hallow | Coated | Swellable | Dissolving

5.5 Clinical Considerations

Chapter 6 details the clinical evidence supporting and practical considerations relevant to microneedling procedures. Regardless of device, treatment principles are similar and involve running needles vertically, horizontally, and diagonally under even pressure. Multiple passes ensure adequate surface coverage with densely packed channels. When performed properly, it is nearly impossible to fully ablate the epidermis, since needles will slip into existing holes if too close together leaving intact surrounding skin.[3,13]

A nuanced treatment plan should account for anatomic location and clinical condition, as tissue thickness and texture varies. Cadaveric studies suggest that facial skin varies from approximately 0.5 mm depth at the upper eyelid to 1.6 to 1.9 mm at the lower nasal sidewall and upper lip. The neck may range from 0.75 to 1.5 mm.[21,22] Penetrating into the papillary and/or reticular dermis, thus, requires different length needles at different locations. Deeper than that (i.e., into the subcutaneous fat) may be no more or in some cases, even less efficacious, as demonstrated in several studies that show similar improvements using 1 and 3 mm depth needles.[16,23] the dense collagen bundles of scarring may warrant a 2 mm setting to traverse a widened, tightly packed dermis.

5.6 Conclusion

Microneedling is an increasingly popular method for cutaneous resurfacing. Mechanical wounding triggers growth factor release and DNA synthesis either through traditional wound healing mechanisms or through a flux in cellular electrical current. Irrespective, these minute injuries appear to upregulate normal epidermal and dermal replication without the production of fibrosis or cicatrix. There are several different types of devices and needles available. Each have advantages and disadvantages so a thorough understanding of your anatomic location, treatment target, and desired outcomes is paramount.

References

[1] Orentreich DS, Orentreich N. Subcutaneous incisionless (subcision) surgery for the correction of depressed scars and wrinkles. Dermatol Surg. 1995; 21(6):543–549

[2] Camirand A, Doucet J. Needle dermabrasion. Aesthetic Plast Surg. 1997; 21(1):48–51

[3] Fernandes D. Minimally invasive percutaneous collagen induction. Oral Maxillofac Surg Clin North Am. 2005; 17(1):51–63, vi

[4] Fabbrocini G, Fardella N, Monfrecola A, Proietti I, Innocenzi D. Acne scarring treatment using skin needling. Clin Exp Dermatol. 2009; 34(8):874–879

[5] Fabbrocini G, De Vita V, Monfrecola A, et al. Percutaneous collagen induction: an effective and safe treatment for postacne scarring in different skin phototypes. J Dermatolog Treat. 2014; 25(2):147–152

[6] Falabella A, Falanga V. Wound Healing. In: Freinkel RK, Woodley DT, eds. The Biology of the Skin. New York, NY: Parethenon; 2001:281–299

[7] McCrudden MT, McAlister E, Courtenay AJ, González-Vázquez P, Singh TR, Donnelly RF. Microneedle applications in improving skin appearance. Exp Dermatol. 2015; 24(8):561–566

[8] Zeitter S, Sikora Z, Jahn S, et al. Microneedling: matching the results of medical needling and repetitive treatments to maximize potential for skin regeneration. Burns. 2014; 40 (5):966–973

[9] Eppley BL, Woodell JE, Higgins J. Platelet quantification and growth factor analysis from platelet-rich plasma: implications for wound healing. Plast Reconstr Surg. 2004; 114(6): 1502–1508

[10] Steed DL. The role of growth factors in wound healing. Surg Clin North Am. 1997; 77(3):575–586

[11] Eming SA. Skin repair—cellular and molecular aspects. In: Bolognia JL, Jorizzo JL, Schaffer JV, eds. Dermatology. 3rd ed. Philadelphia, PA: Elsevier Saunders; 2012:2315–2317

[12] Setterfield L. The Concise Guide to Dermal Needling (expanded Medical Edition). Canada: Acacia Dermacare Inc.; 2013

[13] Liebl H, Kloth LC. Skin cell proliferation stimulated by microneedles. J Am Coll Clin Wound Spec. 2012; 4(1):2–6

[14] El-Domyati M, Barakat M, Awad S, Medhat W, El-Fakahany H, Farag H. Microneedling therapy for atrophic acne scars: an objective evaluation. J Clin Aesthet Dermatol. 2015; 8(7): 36–42

[15] El-Domyati M, Barakat M, Awad S, Medhat W, El-Fakahany H, Farag H. Multiple microneedling sessions for minimally invasive facial rejuvenation: an objective assessment. Int J Dermatol. 2015; 54(12):1361–1369

[16] Aust MC, Fernandes D, Kolokythas P, Kaplan HM, Vogt PM. Percutaneous collagen induction therapy: an alternative treatment for scars, wrinkles, and skin laxity. Plast Reconstr Surg. 2008; 121(4):1421–1429

[17] Jaffe LF. Control of development by steady ionic currents. Fed Proc. 1981; 40(2):125–127

[18] Soltani-Arabshahi R, Wong JW, Duffy KL, Powell DL. Facial allergic granulomatous reaction and systemic hypersensitivity associated with microneedle therapy for skin rejuvenation. JAMA Dermatol. 2014; 150(1):68–72

[19] Serrano G, Almudéver P, Serrano JM, et al. Microneedling dilates the follicular infundibulum and increases transfollicular absorption of liposomal sepia melanin. Clin Cosmet Investig Dermatol. 2015; 8:313–318

[20] Majid I, Sheikh G. Microneedling and its applications in dermatology. PRIME: International Journal of Aesthetics and Anti-Ageing Medicine. 2014

[21] Ha RY, Nojima K, Adams WP, Jr, Brown SA. Analysis of facial skin thickness: defining the relative thickness index. Plast Reconstr Surg. 2005; 115(6):1769–1773

[22] Chopra K, Calva D, Sosin M, et al. A comprehensive examination of topographic thickness of skin in the human face. Aesthet Surg J. 2015; 35(8):1007–1013

[23] Setterfield L. Cosmetic vs. Medical Microneedling. World Aesthetic Medicine Conference, 2009

6
Microneedling: Clinical Applications

Brenda L. Pellicane and Tina S. Alster

Abstract

Microneedling has grown in popularity **over the past several years** for a variety of skin conditions such as alopecia, actinic keratosis, dyschromia, photodamage, and scars. The advantages of microneedling include its cost effectiveness, high clinical efficacy, and excellent safety profile with low complication rate. As a result, microneedling is a valuable alternative or complement to more invasive procedures such as laser skin resurfacing and deep chemical peeling. While microneedling can be used as a stand-alone or in combination with other therapies, further studies to better standardize treatment protocols are needed.

Keywords: microneedling, acne scars, alopecia, actinic keratosis, melasma, skin rejuvenation, striae

Key Points

- **Conditions treated**
  - Nonscarring alopecia.
  - Actinic keratosis.
  - Dyschromia.
  - Rhytides.
  - Scars.
  - Striae.
- **Avoid**
  - Active infection or inflammation (e.g., acne).
- **Prep**
  - Mild cleanser.
  - Topical anesthetic.

- **Technique**
  - Hyaluronic acid gel (or platelet-rich plasma in combination therapy) to facilitate device gliding.
  - Skin traction with perpendicular device tip placement.
  - Cross-hatch microneedling passes.
  - Pinpoint bleeding endpoint.
  - Ice water compression for hemostasis.
- **Postcare**
  - Hydrating gel or cream (e.g., hyaluronic acid or hydrocortisone).
  - Mineral sunblock (SPF 30 +).

6.1 Conditions Treated

6.1.1 Microneedling for Alopecia

Microneedling (MN) has been shown to stimulate stem cells in the bulge region of the hair follicle, release growth factors through platelet activation and wound healing, and induce activation of important genes involved in phases of the hair growth cycle, including vascular endothelial growth factor (VEG-F), B catenin, Wnt3a and Wnt10b.[1] While the use of microneedling in alopecia is fairly limited, early studies show it to be of clinical utility.

Androgenetic Alopecia

Microneedling alone and in combination with topical minoxidil has been used in androgenetic alopecia (AGA) with positive results. A randomized, evaluator-blinded study compared the use of microneedling with 1.5 mm needles and twice-daily minoxidil 5% solution to the use of minoxidil alone in 100 men with mild to moderate androgenetic alopecia. Primary efficacy parameters were assessed at 12 weeks and included change from baseline hair count, patient assessment of hair growth, and investigator assessment of hair growth. The combination treatment group was statistically superior to the minoxidil only group in all three efficacy measures.[2]

A subsequent case series of four male patients with stable AGA being treated with finasteride and minoxidil 5% solution received a series of 15 microneedling treatments over a 6-month period. Therapy with the finasteride and minoxidil was ongoing. Microneedling was performed on betadine-prepped scalp using a Dermaroller 1.5 mm with mild erythema as the clinical endpoint. After 8 to 10 sessions, new hair growth was observed in all four patients. Patient satisfaction ranged from 50 to 75% and results were sustained at 18 months follow-up.[3]

A study comparing topical minoxidil to monthly sessions of combined platelet-rich plasma mesotherapy and scalp micro-needling showed comparable results with regard to improvement of hair density; however, onset was significantly faster with minoxidil (▶ Fig. 6.1).[4]

Alopecia Areata

Alopecia areata is an autoimmune inflammatory condition affecting hair follicles, which leads to usually discrete or less often diffuse patches of hair loss. Standard treatment with topical and intralesional corticosteroids is often ineffective or provides only temporary amelioration. Microneedling was shown to be effective in inducing hair growth in two patients with alopecia areata who had failed previous treatment with intralesional triacminolone acetonide, topical steroids, and minoxidil 5% lotion.[5] Triamcinolone acetonide (10 mg/mL) was applied to the scalp both before and after microneedling using a Dermaroller with 1.5 mm needles. Three treatments were performed at 3-week intervals. Anesthesia was not necessary as the patients reported the procedure as painless. The investigators used pinpoint bleeding as their clinical end point and noted progressive improvement after each session. Three weeks following the final

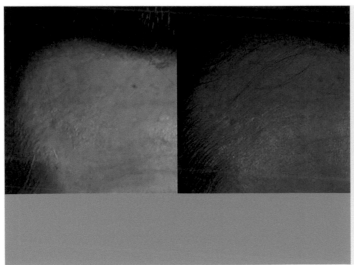

Fig. 6.1 Androgenic alopecia at baseline (left) and 3 months after third monthly microneedling session without concomitant topical therapy (right).

treatment, regrowth was considered excellent with results maintained 3 months posttreatment. The authors proposed that microneedling facilitated uniform and enhanced absorption of triamcinolone acetonide that could mitigate steroid-associated atrophy and limit the discomfort experienced with intralesional therapies.

6.1.2 Microneedling for Actinic Keratoses

Photodynamic therapy (PDT) is an approved effective treatment for treatment of actinic keratoses (AKs). Additionally, PDT has demonstrated cosmetic benefits. The effects of PDT are dose and time dependent and contingent, in part, on penetration of the photosensitizing agent. The stratum corneum (SC) is the main barrier to drug absorption. Physical pretreatment of the skin facilitates local uptake and is recommended to optimize results.[6] Studies showing increased protoporphyrin IX (PPIX) fluorescence suggest that microneedling prior to and following application of photosensitizers, such as methyl aminolevulinate (MAL) and delta amino levulinic acid (ALA), enhance their absorption.[7]

Clementoni et al showed statistically significant improvement in global photoaging scores in 21 patients treated with combination red light and broadband pulsed light following microneedling at 0.3 mm depth than 1 hour incubation with 5-ALA.[8] However, lack of controls made it impossible to determine whether the clinical improvement was due to the combination of techniques or the PDT alone.

A split-face study compared conventional MAL–PDT preceded by curettage on one facial half to MAL–PDT followed by microneedling on the contralateral side.[9] After a 90-minute incubation, skin was irradiated with red LED. Side effects were more common, intense, and persisted longer on the side treated with a 1.5 mm microneedling device. No significant difference in actinic keratoses clearance rate between facial halves was noted, yet the microneedling-assisted PDT side had superior cosmetic results with greater improvement in mottled pigmentation, roughness, coarse wrinkles, fine lines and sallowness. The authors attributed the enhanced cosmetic improvement to better tissue delivery of the MAL and to the microneedle-induced wound healing response.

Another split-face study demonstrated both a greater decrease in mean percentage of actinic keratoses and increased cosmetic benefit on the side treated with microneedling prior to PDT compared to the standard PDT-treated side alone.[10] Microneedling was performed with a mechanical stamp style device at 0.5 mm. The skin was incubated with ALA for 1 hour prior to using the BLU U blue light for 1,000 seconds. It was unclear whether the cosmetic improvement resulted from the microneedling procedure itself, deeper penetration of the photosensitizer, or both.

A randomized study of 33 individuals with actinic keratoses revealed that 20 minute ALA incubation time following a microneedle roller (200 µm) with 1,000 seconds blue light exposure (total fluence 10 J/cm^2) was superior to a 10 minute ALA incubation time.[11] Average actinic keratosis clearance was 76% with the 20 minute ALA incubation and 43% with the 10 minute ALA incubation, the latter not meeting statistical significance. The expedited 20-minute ALA incubation protocol mirrored the clinical efficacy typically achieved with conventional 1 hour

ALA incubation time, thereby providing a suitable alternative to the time burden of standard PDT treatment.

While studies support the use of microneedling in conjunction with PDT, whether for treatment of actinic keratoses or improved cosmesis, it is important to note that other techniques can also facilitate absorption of photosensitizers. Bay et al found that the protoporphyrin IX accumulation was most enhanced following pretreatment with ablative fractional laser (10,600-nm fractional carbon dioxide [CO_2]), followed by microdermabrasion, microneedling (0.2 mm Dermaroller) and curettage.[12] In clinical practice, however, practicality must be considered given that microneedling is minimally painful, significantly less expensive, faster to perform, and low downtime versus ablative fractionated laser treatment.

Improved efficacy of PDT has significant implications and may be particularly useful in organ transplant recipients. This population is immunosuppressed and has a substantially higher incidence of actinic keratoses compared to immunocompetent individuals. A study of 12 transplant recipients with actinic keratoses resistant to classical PDT showed a high clearance rate and low risk of recurrence after a series of three PDT treatments in which patients were pretreated with microneedling with a depth of 0.5 mm.[13]

6.1.3 Microneedling for Dyspigmentation (▶ Fig. 6.2a, b)

Melasma

Melasma is a common pigmentary disorder that is chronic and often recalcitrant to treatment. Photoprotection, topical treatments, chemical peels, and lasers have been used to treat melasma with varying results. Microneedling has been used with success to enhance melasma treatment results, although the mechanism of skin lightening is not yet well established. A study by Fabbrocini et al compared the use of microneedling (Dermaroller 0.5 mm) followed by application of a depigmenting serum (containing rucinol and sophora-alpha) on one side of the face with depigmenting serum alone on the contralateral side. Two treatments were performed at 1-month intervals. After each treatment, patients used a home roller device (Dermaroller-Model C8, 0.13 mm needle length) once-daily followed immediately by application of the depigmenting serum. Sunscreen was used on both sides of the face. Compared to the facial half treated with depigmenting serum alone, the combination therapy side had a statistically significant reduction in pigmentation and improved luminosity index.[14]

A study of 22 patients with melasma recalcitrant to topical therapy and sunscreen were treated with two sessions of microneedling using a 1.5 mm Dermaroller at 1-month intervals. Twenty-four hours after the procedure, patients initiated daily application of a topical lightening agent (0.05% tretinoin + 4% hydroquinone + 1% fluocinolone acetonide) and SPF 60 sunscreen. The treatment was well-tolerated, and all patients responded and were satisfied with their clinical results.[15]

Tranexamic acid (TA), a synthetic derivative of the amino acid lysine, is primarily used for its antihemorrhagic and antifibrinolytic properties in a surgical setting.[16] Topical TA has been found to decrease melanocyte tyrosinase activity through inhibition of ultraviolet (UV)-induced plasmin activity in keratinocytes.[17] Intradermal microinjections have been used as a

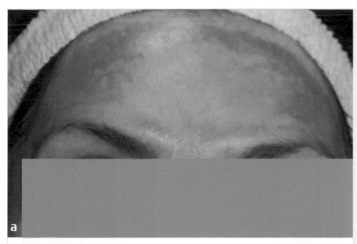

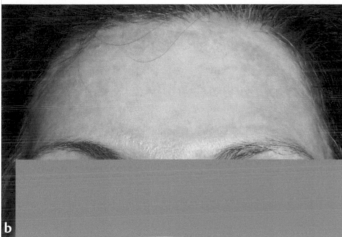

Fig. 6.2 Melasma on the forehead at (a) baseline and (b) 6 months after one microneedling session and daily posttreatment use of mineral SPF 50 sunblock and topical vitamin C serum.

treatment for melasma.[18] A study comparing microinjections of TA with topical TA both preceded and followed by at 1.5 mm microneedling (TA 4 mg/mL; Arm 1 with maximum 8 mg injected into a single area vs. Arm 2 with 4 to 5 cycles of 0.5 to 1 mL TA applied topically during needling) showed a better therapeutic response in the microneedling group, which was attributed to deeper and more uniform delivery of the TA.[19]

Microneedling has also been shown to augment the response of melasma to laser treatment. A split-face study compared Q-switched (QS) Nd:YAG followed immediately by microneedling and vitamin C application to QS Nd:YAG alone for a series of four monthly treatments.[20] The combination treatment side demonstrated significantly better treatment response and greater improvement in MASI (Melasma Area Severity Index) scores. It was proposed that the QS Nd:YAG laser increased dermal circulation and thereby enhanced the microneedling mechanical effect and facilitated vitamin C penetration. It is important to note, however, that the risk of adverse events (particularly dermatitis) increases with the concomitant use of lasers and/or microneedling with topical products that are not intended for intradermal application.

Periorbital Melanosis

Microneedling has been used to successfully treat periorbital melanosis, a multifactorial condition often recalcitrant to treatment. Infraorbital dark circles were successfully treated in 13 women using a combination of microneedling followed by application of 10% trichloroacetic acid (TCA) for 5 minutes. Significant aesthetic improvement was seen in nearly all patients.[21]

A case report using DermaFrac (Genesis Biosystems), which combines microneedling and simultaneous vacuum-assisted infusion of a serum, showed significant improvement of periorbital melanosis in an Indian male patient.[22] A total of 12 treatments were performed at 2-week intervals with application of either an "antiaging serum" or "lightening serum" (containing kojic acid). The favorable results reported may have been due to increased hydration and stimulation of new collagen and elastin reducing visibility of dermal pigment and blood vessels.

6.1.4 Microneedling for Skin Rejuvenation (▶ Fig. 6.3a, b)

Microneedling therapy has been successfully used as a minimally invasive treatment for skin aging.[23,24] A study of 10 patients treated with six microneedling sessions at 2-week intervals showed histologic and clinical evidence of efficacy.[25] Biopsy specimens at 3 months confirmed epidermal acanthosis with rete ridge development. Interestingly, the total elastin content dropped, likely

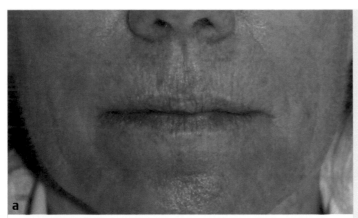
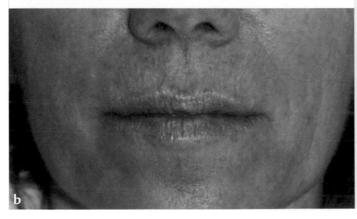

Fig. 6.3 Perioral rhytides at (a) baseline and (b) 3 months after one microneedling session.

because solar elastotic material decreased while tropoelastin, a precursor to elastin, increased. This observation suggests that histology obtained at an early 3-month time point failed to capture the full tissue regeneration response and subsequent biopsies might have shown an overall rise in elastin content as the precursor tropoelastin aggregates into mature, well-organized rather than UV-irradiated fibers. New synthesis of collagen types I, III, and VII was also demonstrated. Results for collagen content were statistically significant at 3 months posttreatment and anticipated to improve further during the 1 year neocollagenesis process.[26] The collagen formed in the early phases of wound healing is type III then gradually replaced by collagen I, which remains in the area for 5 to 7 years.[23] Similar results were achieved in a retrospective analysis of 480 patients who received a series of one to four treatments. Increased collagen, in a normal lattice pattern, was observed 6 months posttreatment and a 40% increase in epidermal thickening was evident at 1 year. This study also found increase in elastic fibers at the later 6-month time points.[27]

Microneedling has been utilized for hand rejuvenation, an increasingly popular area of concern. An initial feasibility study showed improved skin texture, skin tightening, and dermal neovascularization without dyspigmentation of dorsal hand skin after one microneedling treatment (depth unspecified).[28] Microneedling also successfully treated the aging neck in eight patients. Multiple modalities were used to assess efficacy including photographs, ultrasonographic images, and silicone rubber microrelief impressions. Two treatments led to a reduction in wrinkle severity grade in almost 90% of

the patients.[29] Similarly, two sessions of microneedling of the upper lip showed marked reduction in wrinkle severity as assessed by photography and computer analysis of silicone rubber impressions of the wrinkles.[30]

6.1.5 Microneedling for Scars

Numerous treatments exist for scar revision and often the best cosmetic outcomes are achieved by combining therapies.[31,32]

Acne Scars (▶ Fig. 6.4a, b)

Acne is one of the most common skin conditions and frequently leads to scarring caused by inflammation destroying underlying dermal support structures. The result is atrophic scars, which are commonly classified as ice pick, rolling, or box car.[33] Numerous treatment modalities have been used to treat acne scars. Microneedling has a favorable treatment profile, since it is minimally invasive, has a relatively rapid recovery time with a low risk of postinflammatory hyperpigmentation (PIH), is comparatively inexpensive, and can be used safely across a wide range of skin phototypes.[34,35,36] The procedure disrupts fibrotic strands tethering the scars to the dermis[37] and induces neoangiogenesis and neocollagenesis through induction of the wound-healing cascade.[38]

Multiple studies have demonstrated both clinical and histological improvement of acne scarring after microneedling treatment. Using histological analysis, El-Domyati et al demonstrated a significant increase in epidermal thickening, collagen I, III, VII, and tropoelastin.[39] Statistically significant improvement was demonstrated in scar severity, skin texture, and patient satisfaction. Greater clinical improvement

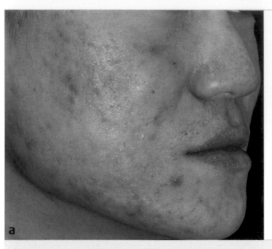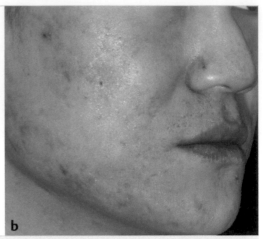

Fig. 6.4 Atrophic facial acne scars at **(a)** baseline and **(b)** 6 months after three microneedling sessions at monthly intervals.

was seen in rolling and box car scars than in ice pick scars.

The use of nonablative fractional erbium laser 1,340 nm for atrophic acne scars was compared with the use of microneedling (Dr. Roller, 2 mm needles) in 46 patients randomized to receive three monthly sessions of either laser or microneedling.[40] Both groups showed significant clinical improvement with no statistically significant clinical difference between treatment groups; however, the laser-treated participants exhibited longer duration of erythema (median of 3 vs. 1 day) and 13.6% of patients had hyperpigmentation. No patients in the microneedling-treated group experienced dyspigmentation. While a higher proportion of laser-treated patients reported noticeable improvement after one treatment, 100% of both groups perceived improvement after the second treatment session.[40]

Another comparison study of 30 patients with atrophic acne scars used a fractional Er:YAG laser on one facial half and microneedling (Dermapen, 12 needles, 2 mm depth) on the contralateral facial half.[41] While both modalities induced noticeable clinical and histological improvement at

3 months after a series of five monthly treatments, significantly better clinical results were observed in fractional Er:YAG laser irradiated areas than in microneedled areas (70 vs. 30%, respectively). The microneedled areas healed at a significantly faster rate.

Recent studies suggest that clinical results may be enhanced by the use of additional treatments delivered in tandem. Microneedling followed immediately by 20% TCA application or 1540 nm nonablative fractionated laser was superior to either treatment alone.[42] Similarly, the combined use of microneedling with 35% glycolic acid peels showed superior results to microneedling in isolation.[43] In another study, improvement in acne scarring was achieved with alternating sessions of microneedling and 15% TCA peels performed at 2 week intervals; however, 6% of patients developed PIH.[44]

PRP in combination with microneedling has also been shown to increase efficacy of acne scar treatment above and beyond microneedling alone (Chapter 9).[45,46] While PRP may improve cosmetic outcomes, the clinical significance of supplemental treatment should be weighed against the increased expense, since PRP often doubles procedural costs.

Other Scars (▶ Fig. 6.5a, b)

Varicella scars clinically mimic atrophic acne scars and not surprisingly, have been effectively treated with microneedling. A 15-year-old girl with Fitzpatrick skin phototype V and a history of childhood varicella showed significant scar improvement after three monthly microneedling sessions (cylindrical roller, 1.5 mm needles) without complications.[47]

Microneedling has also been successful in the treatment of burn scars with marked clinical and histological improvement. A series of 16 patients with mature burn scars (at least 2 years postinjury) received one to four microneedling treatments (Medical Roll-CIT, depth unspecified).[48] Scars were pretreated with vitamin A (retinyl palmitate) and vitamin C (ascorbyl tetraisopalmitate) creams for a minimum of one month prior to microneedling and also between treatment sessions. Patients rated clinical improvement as a mean of 80% or better on a visual analog scale. Histological analysis one year post-therapy revealed increased collagen and elastin deposition, 45% thickening of the stratum spinosum with normal rete ridges, and normalization of the reticular dermis collagen-elastin matrix.

Repigmentation of large hypopigmented scars has not been effective with microneedling as a sole treatment.[49] The use of a topical noncultured autologous skin cell suspension in combination with microneedling, however, showed improvement of melanin index scores when compared to microneedling alone.[50]

Striae

Striae are a common and distressing skin condition for which no fully effective treatments exist to date.[51] One session of microneedling in 22 women resulted in improved skin texture, skin tightening, and dermal neovascularization at 6 months posttreatment with histology demonstrating increased collagen I and elastin content.[52] Park and colleagues similarly demonstrated clinical

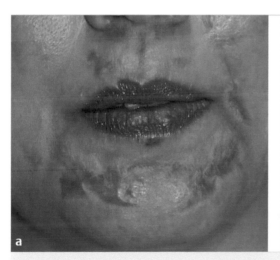
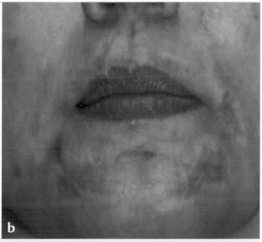

Fig. 6.5 Facial burn scars at (a) baseline and (b) 3 months after two microneedling sessions at 1-month intervals.

improvement of striae rubra and alba in a pilot study.[53]

Khater et al also demonstrated the superior clinical effect of microneedling over fractional CO_2 laser for striae.[54] Patients' abdomens and lower limbs were treated with either needling therapy (1.5 mm needle length) or fractional CO_2 laser every month for three sessions. While both groups showed increased epidermal thickness and fibroblasts 6 months after treatment, 90% of the microneedle-treated patients showed clinical improvement compared to 50% of the laser-treated patients. Higher patient satisfaction with significantly faster healing and fewer side effects were reported in the group treated with microneedling. In another study, microneedling was similarly found to be superior to microdermabrasion with sonophoresis.[55]

6.2 Microneedling: Technical and Clinical Considerations

6.2.1 Technical Considerations

The original microneedling devices consisted of evenly distributed needles affixed to a drum-shaped roller. Most microneedling publications to date involved the use of these roller devices. In recent years, microneedling devices have evolved to include corded and battery-powered pens with disposable tips containing 12 to 36 needles.[24,56] Automated pen devices offer variability of needle depth (0.25 to 3.0 mm) with a single cartridge and are small enough to treat areas difficult to access by a roller device. In addition to their enhanced sterility and maneuverability, they can more effectively and reliably penetrate into the deeper dermis to produce improved clinical outcomes (Chapter 5).

6.2.2 Treatment Preparation (▶ Fig. 6.6)

Microneedling is a simple, office-based procedure, typically ranging in duration from 5 to 15 minutes depending on the size of the area to be treated. Some practitioners advocate pretreatment for a minimum of three weeks with topical vitamins A and C due to their effects on skin cell proliferation and differentiation (vitamin A) and neocollagenesis (vitamin C).[29,57] While use of shallow needle lengths (< 0.5 mm) does not necessitate use of topical anesthesia, it is often applied for more aggressive microneedling procedures. Acne and other scars typically require needle lengths of 1.5 to 2.0 mm, whereas skin rejuvenation may only require needles of 0.5 to 1.0 mm considering the skin thickness in different anatomic regions (Chapter 5).[58] In these latter cases, topical anesthesia is applied to cleaned skin for 15 to 60 minutes depending on the anesthetic used, area being treated and needle depth used.

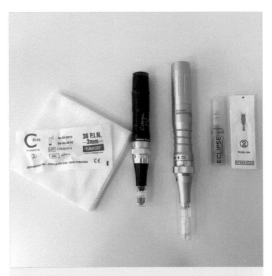

Fig. 6.6 Microneedling devices, needle tips, and gliding gel.

6.2.3 Operative Technique (▶ Fig. 6.7 and ▶ Fig. 6.8)

After the topical anesthetic is removed, prep the skin with an antiseptic. Gentle traction of the skin while applying the microneedling device perpendicular to the surface assists the smooth, vertical delivery of microneedles into the dermis. For lax skin areas such as the upper lip or cheeks, a gauze roll or gloved finger can be placed between the teeth and buccal mucosa for additional support. A topical serum (e.g., hyaluronic acid or PRP in the case of combination therapy) is typically applied to the treatment areas in order to facilitate gliding of the device across the skin and to prevent untoward injury to the overlying epidermis. Multiple passes of the device are applied over the treatment area in a multidirectional or cross-hatching pattern until lesional effacement and/or pinpoint bleeding is observed. Some practitioners also use circular motions. Sterile ice water or saline-soaked sterile gauze is used to remove excess blood and to achieve hemostasis.

Microneedling Set-Up

- Microneedling device and disposable tip.
- Disposable gloves.
- Hyaluronic acid gel.
- Ice water in bowl.
- 4 × 4 gauze.
- Topical anesthetic.

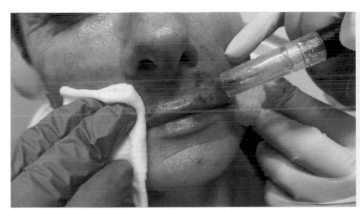

Fig. 6.7 Gentle traction is applied while the microneedle tip is held perpendicular to the skin's surface in order to facilitate smooth delivery of microneedles to the skin in a multi-directional (or crosshatching) pattern.

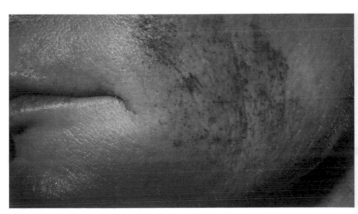

Fig. 6.8 Pinpoint bleeding is used as a visual endpoint of treatment. Hemostasis is achieved with application of ice water-soaked sterile gauze.

6.2.4 Posttreatment Care

A thin layer of hyaluronic acid gel or a topical hydrocortisone-containing balm can be applied immediately after the treatment. Posttreatment skin care consists of gentle cleansing with a mild soap followed by application of a nonallergenic moisturizing cream or topical hydrocortisone several times daily. It is important to avoid application of substances that are not approved for intradermal use due to the possibility of dermatitis or granuloma formation, since microneedle-induced channels have been reported to remain open for several hours posttreatment.[59] The use of a mineral (nonchemical) sunblock with SPF 30 or higher is advocated in order to avoid unwanted posttreatment dyspigmentation. Makeup application can be initiated 2 days posttreatment and regular (active) skin care products can be resumed in 5 to 7 days (when erythema has resolved).

Additional treatment sessions are generally recommended at monthly, or less commonly biweekly, time intervals until the desired clinical results are achieved. Some patients elect to receive maintenance treatment sessions on an annual or semiannual basis in order to enhance their cosmetic outcomes.[24,58]

6.3 Conclusion

Microneedling has become an integral part of the daily treatment algorithm for the treatment of alopecia, actinic keratosis, dyschromia, photodamage, and scars. Its excellent safety profile, high clinical efficacy, and fast posttreatment recovery make microneedling a valuable alternative to more invasive procedures. Additional studies are needed to define specific treatment protocols for these and other conditions to improve clinical practice.

References

[1] Kim YS, Jeong KH, Kim JE, Woo YJ, Kim BJ, Kang H. Repeated microneedle stimulation induces enhanced hair growth in a murine model. Ann Dermatol. 2016; 28(5):586–592

[2] Dhurat R, Sukesh M, Avhad G, Dandale A, Pal A, Pund P. A randomized evaluator blinded study of effect of microneedling in androgenetic alopecia: a pilot study. Int J Trichology. 2013; 5(1):6–11

[3] Dhurat R, Mathapati S. Response to microneedling treatment in men with androgenetic alopecia who failed to respond to conventional therapy. Indian J Dermatol. 2015; 60(3):260–263

[4] Farid CI, Abdelmaksoud RA. Platelet-rich plasma microneedling versus 5% topical minoxidil in the treatment of patterned hair loss. J Egyptian Women Dermatol Society. 2016; 13(1):29–36

[5] Chandrashekar B, Yepuri V, Mysore V. Alopecia areata-successful outcome with microneedling and triamcinolone acetonide. J Cutan Aesthet Surg. 2014; 7(1):63–64

[6] Christensen E, Warloe T, Kroon S, et al. Norwegian Photodynamic Therapy (PDT) Group. Guidelines for practical use of MAL-PDT in non-melanoma skin cancer. J Eur Acad Dermatol Venereol. 2010; 24(5):505–512

[7] Mikolajewska P, Donnelly RF, Garland MJ, et al. Microneedle pre-treatment of human skin improves 5-aminolevulininc acid (ALA)- and 5-aminolevulinic acid methyl ester (MAL)-induced PpIX production for topical photodynamic therapy without increase in pain or erythema. Pharm Res. 2010; 27 (10):2213–2220

[8] Clementoni MT, B-Roscher M, Munavalli GS. Photodynamic photorejuvenation of the face with a combination of microneedling, red light, and broadband pulsed light. Lasers Surg Med. 2010; 42(2):150–159

[9] Torezan L, Chaves Y, Niwa A, Sanches JA, Jr, Festa-Neto C, Szeimies RM. A pilot split-face study comparing conventional methyl aminolevulinate-photodynamic therapy (PDT) with microneedling-assisted PDT on actinically damaged skin. Dermatol Surg. 2013; 39(8):1197–1201

[10] Spencer JM, Freeman SA. Microneedling prior to levulan PDT for the treatment of actinic keratoses: a split-face, blinded trial. J Drugs Dermatol. 2016; 15(9):1072–1074

[11] Petukhova TA, Hassoun LA, Foolad N, Barath M, Sivamani RK. Effect of expedited microneedle-assisted photodynamic therapy for field treatment of actinic keratoses: a randomized clinical trial. JAMA Dermatol. 2017; 153(7):637–643

[12] Bay C, Lerche CM, Ferrick B, Philipsen PA, Togsverd-Bo K, Haedersdal M. Comparison of physical pretreatment regimens to enhance protoporphyrin IX uptake in photodynamic therapy: a randomized clinical trial. JAMA Dermatol. 2017; 153(4):270–278

[13] Bencini PL, Galimberti MG, Pellacani G, Longo C. Application of photodynamic therapy combined with pre-illumination microneedling in the treatment of actinic keratosis in organ transplant recipients. Br J Dermatol. 2012; 167(5):1193–1194

[14] Fabbrocini G, De Vita V, Fardella N, et al. Skin needling to enhance depigmenting serum penetration in the treatment of melasma. Plast Surg Int. 2011; 2011:158241

[15] Lima EdeA. Microneedling in facial recalcitrant melasma: report of a series of 22 cases. An Bras Dermatol. 2015; 90(6): 919–921

[16] Dunn CJ, Goa KL. Tranexamic acid: a review of its use in surgery and other indications. Drugs. 1999; 57(6):1005–1032

[17] Maeda K, Naganuma M. Topical trans-4-aminomethylcyclohexanecarboxylic acid prevents ultraviolet radiation-induced

pigmentation. J Photochem Photobiol B. 1998; 47(2–3): 136–141

[18] Lee JH, Park JG, Lim SH, et al. Localized intradermal microinjection of tranexamic acid for treatment of melasma in Asian patients: a preliminary clinical trial. Dermatol Surg. 2006; 32 (5):626–631

[19] Budamakuntla L, Loganathan E, Suresh DH, et al. A randomised, open-label, comparative study of tranexamic acid microinjections and tranexamic acid with microneedling in patients with melasma. J Cutan Aesthet Surg. 2013; 6(3): 139–143

[20] Ustuner P, Balevi A, Ozdemir M. A split-face, investigator-blinded comparative study on the efficacy and safety of Q-switched Nd:YAG laser plus microneedling with vitamin C versus Q-switched Nd:YAG laser for the treatment of recalcitrant melasma. J Cosmet Laser Ther. 2017; 19(7):383–390

[21] Kontochristopoulos G, Kouris A, Platsidaki E, Markantoni V, Gerodimou M, Antoniou C. Combination of microneedling and 10% trichloroacetic acid peels in the management of infraorbital dark circles. J Cosmet Laser Ther. 2016; 18(5):289–292

[22] Sahni K, Kassir M. Dermafrac™: an innovative new treatment for periorbital melanosis in a dark-skinned male patient. J Cutan Aesthet Surg. 2013; 6(3):158–160

[23] Fernandes D, Signorini M. Combating photoaging with percutaneous collagen induction. Clin Dermatol. 2008; 26(2): 192–199

[24] Alster TS, Graham PM. Microneedling: a review and practical guide. Dermatol Surg. 2018; 44:397–404

[25] El-Domyati M, Barakat M, Awad S, Medhat W, El-Fakahany H, Farag H. Multiple microneedling sessions for minimally invasive facial rejuvenation: an objective assessment. Int J Dermatol. 2015; 54(12):1361–1369

[26] Fernandes D. Minimally invasive percutaneous collagen induction. Oral Maxillofac Surg Clin North Am. 2005, 17(1): 51–63, vi

[27] Aust MC, Fernandes D, Kolokythas P, Kaplan HM, Vogt PM. Percutaneous collagen induction therapy: an alternative treatment for scars, wrinkles, and skin laxity. Plast Reconstr Surg. 2008; 121(4):1421–1429

[28] Lee HJ, Lee EG, Kang S, Sung JH, Chung HM, Kim DH. Efficacy of microneedling plus human stem cell conditioned medium for skin rejuvenation: a randomized, controlled, blinded split-face study. Ann Dermatol. 2014; 26(5):584–591

[29] Aust M, Knobloch K, Gohritz A, Vogt PM, Fernandes D. Percutaneous collagen induction therapy for hand rejuvenation. Plast Reconstr Surg. 2010; 126(4):203e–204e

[30] Fabbrocini G, De Vita V, Di Costanzo L, et al. Skin needling in the treatment of the aging neck. Skinmed. 2011; 9(6): 347–351

[31] Fabbrocini G, De Vita V, Pastore F, et al. Collagen induction therapy for the treatment of upper lip wrinkles. J Dermatolog Treat. 2012; 23(2):144–152

[32] Eilers RE, Jr, Ross EV, Cohen JL, Ortiz AE. A combination approach to surgical scars. Dermatol Surg. 2016; 42 Suppl 2: S150–S156

[33] Sobanko JF, Alster TS. Management of acne scarring, part I: a comparative review of laser surgical approaches. Am J Clin Dermatol. 2012; 13(5):319–330

[34] Jacob CI, Dover JS, Kaminer MS. Acne scarring: a classification system and review of treatment options. J Am Acad Dermatol. 2001; 45(1):109–117

[35] Fabbrocini G, De Vita V, Monfrecola A, et al. Percutaneous collagen induction: an effective and safe treatment for post-acne scarring in different skin phototypes. J Dermatolog Treat. 2014; 25(2):147–152

[36] Dogra S, Yadav S, Sarangal R. Microneedling for acne scars in Asian skin type: an effective low cost treatment modality. J Cosmet Dermatol. 2014; 13(3):180–187

[37] Fabbrocini G, Fardella N, Monfrecola A, Proietti I, Innocenzi D. Acne scarring treatment using skin needling. Clin Exp Dermatol. 2009; 34(8):874–879

[38] Liebl H, Kloth LC. Skin cell proliferation stimulated by microneedles. J Am Coll Clin Wound Spec. 2012; 4(1):2–6

[39] El-Domyati M, Barakat M, Awad S, Medhat W, El-Fakahany H, Farag H. Microneedling therapy for atrophic acne scars: an objective evaluation. J Clin Aesthet Dermatol. 2015; 8(7):36–42

[40] Cachafeiro T, Escobar G, Maldonado G, Cestari T, Corleta O. Comparison of nonablative fractional erbium laser 1,340 nm and microneedling for the treatment of atrophic acne scars: a randomized clinical trial. Dermatol Surg. 2016; 42(2):232–241

[41] Osman MA, Shokeir HA, Fawzy MM. Fractional erbium-doped yttrium aluminum garnet laser versus microneedling in treatment of atrophic acne scars: a randomized split-face clinical study. Dermatol Surg. 2017; 43 Suppl 1:S47–S56

[42] Leheta TM, Abdel Hay RM, Hegazy RA, El Garem YF. Do combined alternating sessions of 1540 nm nonablative fractional laser and percutaneous collagen induction with trichloroacetic acid 20% show better results than each individual modality in the treatment of atrophic acne scars? A randomized controlled trial. J Dermatolog Treat. 2014; 25(2):137–141

[43] Sharad J. Combination of microneedling and glycolic acid peels for the treatment of acne scars in dark skin. J Cosmet Dermatol. 2011; 10(4):317–323

[44] Garg S, Baveja S. Combination therapy in the management of atrophic acne scars. J Cutan Aesthet Surg. 2014; 7(1):18–23

[45] Asif M, Kanodia S, Singh K. Combined autologous platelet-rich plasma with microneedling verses microneedling with distilled water in the treatment of atrophic acne scars: a concurrent split-face study. J Cosmet Dermatol. 2016; 15(4): 434–443

[46] Ibrahim ZA, El-Ashmawy AA, Shora OA. Therapeutic effect of microneedling and autologous platelet-rich plasma in the treatment of atrophic scars: A randomized study. J Cosmet Dermatol. 2017; 16(3):388–399

[47] Costa IM, Costa MC. Microneedling for varicella scars in a dark-skinned teenager. Dermatol Surg. 2014; 40(3):333–334

[48] Aust MC, Knobloch K, Reimers K, et al. Percutaneous collagen induction therapy: an alternative treatment for burn scars. Burns. 2010; 36(6):836–843

[49] Aust MC, Reimers K, Repenning C, et al. Percutaneous collagen induction: minimally invasive skin rejuvenation without risk of hyperpigmentation-fact or fiction? Plast Reconstr Surg. 2008; 122(5):1553–1563

[50] Busch KH, Bender R, Walezko N, Aziz H, Altintas MA, Aust MC. Combination of medical needling and non-cultured autologous skin cell transplantation (ReNovaCell) for repigmentation of hypopigmented burn scars. Burns. 2016; 42(7): 1556–1566

[51] Alster TS, Greenberg HL. Laser treatment of scars and striae. In: Kauvar ANB, Hruza G, eds. Principles and Practices in Cutaneous Laser Surgery. New York, NY: Taylor & Francis; 2005:619–635

[52] Aust MC, Knobloch K, Vogt PM. Percutaneous collagen induction therapy as a novel therapeutic option for Striae distensae. Plast Reconstr Surg. 2010; 126(4):219e–220e

[53] Park KY, Kim HK, Kim SE, Kim BJ, Kim MN. Treatment of striae distensae using needling therapy: a pilot study. Dermatol Surg. 2012; 38(11):1823–1828

[54] Khater MH, Khattab FM, Abdelhaleem MR. Treatment of striae distensae with needling therapy versus CO2 fractional laser. J Cosmet Laser Ther. 2016; 18(2):75–79

[55] Nassar A, Ghomey S, El Gohary Y, El-Desoky F. Treatment of striae distensae with needling therapy versus microdermabrasion with sonophoresis. J Cosmet Laser Ther. 2016; 18(6): 330–334

[56] Hashim PW, Levy Z, Cohen JL, Goldenberg G. Microneedling therapy with and without platelet-rich plasma. Cutis. 2017; 99(4):239–242

[57] Fernandes D. Percutaneous collagen induction: an alternative to laser resurfacing. Aesthet Surg J. 2002; 22(3):307–309

[58] Singh A, Yadav S. Microneedling: advances and widening horizons. Indian Dermatol Online J. 2016; 7(4):244–254

[59] Bal S, Kruithof AC, Liebl H, et al. In vivo visualization of micro-needle conduits in human skin using laser scanning microscopy. Laser Phys Lett. 2010; 7(3):242–246

7
Microneedling and Radiofrequency

Chatchadaporn Chunharas, Douglas C. Wu, and Mitchel P. Goldman

Abstract

Microneedling radiofrequency is safe and effective procedure with minimal downtime and low risk of postinflammatory hyperpigmentation. The information reviewed in this chapter demonstrates that microneedling with radiofrequency can significantly improve various skin conditions such as acne, acne scars, fine lines and wrinkles, primary axillary hyperhidrosis, striae distensae, and rosacea. The treatment is appropriate for all skin types, and offers an alternative treatment for patients with darker skin.

Keywords: microneedling radiofrequency, fractional radiofrequency, sublative fractional radiofrequency, bipolar fractional radiofrequency, acne, acne scar, skin rejuvenation, wrinkle, primary axillary hyperhidrosis, rosacea, striae distensae

Key Points

- Acne scar is the most common indication for microneedling radiofrequency (MRF) treatment. Combination of MRF with other modalities, such as diode laser bipolar radiofrequency or subcision, has been proven effective. Also, favorable results can be achieved by combining fractionated and unfractionated ablative and non-ablative laser, vascular lasers, pigment lasers, focused ultrasound, and injectable soft-tissue fillers.
- MRF shows a promised benefit for controlling active acne. The improvement of acne might be due to the reduction in some sebaceous glands and reduction in perifolliculitis.
- Improvement of a sign of photodamage, skin laxity, texture, fine lines, and wrinkles are observed in multiple studies across different skin types and ethnicity. MRF can be used for facial rejuvenation, as well as neck laxity. MRF treatment might provide a nonsurgical option for the treatment of facial skin laxity in patients.
- MRF is also beneficial in other difficult to treat skin condition such as primary axillary hyperhidrosis, rosacea, and striae distensae.
- Adverse events of MRF are limited to mild pain, transient erythema or edema, and rarely epidermal atrophy after the procedure. Fewer patients demonstrate postinflammatory hyperpigmentation compared to ablative and non-ablative laser resurfacing. Skin depressions have been reported. It can be avoided by optimal contact of the hand piece to the skin and using the appropriate energy.

7.1 Radiofrequency (RF)

Radiofrequency (RF) is the term given to any alternating electrical current that, if applied to an antenna, creates an electromagnetic field, which propagates through space and time in the surrounding area. The radiofrequency spectrum can be divided into bands ranging from very low frequency (3–30 kHz) to extremely high frequency (30–300 GHz). Energy generated can be transmitted and applied directly to tissues, which absorb and even retransmit the current. Because RF radiation has a short wavelength, it interacts with polar molecules such as water, amino acids, and nucleic acids, producing a molecular vibration that is converted to thermal energy. This energy transmission changes according to the resistance of the tissue. Therefore, RF delivers heat energy to tissues nonspecifically. This process is unlike lasers, which depend on chromophores that absorb optical energy converting it to heat.[1] RF does not affect skin color and so it can be used safely on various skin types.

7.2 Microneedling

Microneedling is a minimally invasive procedure using fine needles to puncture the epidermis. Needling alone has proved beneficial to the skin, improving blood flow and wound healing in an animal flap model.[2] Fernandes developed the dermaroller mounted with tiny needles to create the microwounds in the skin.[3] Microneedling devices can be used to treat various skin conditions including acne and other scars, facial rejuvenation, dyspigmentation, alopecia, and hyperhidrosis.

7.3 Microneedling RF (MRF)

A pilot study by Hantash and colleagues was the first clinical application of Microneedling RF (MRF). Histologic analyses of treated skin excised from subsequent abdominoplasty or facelift procedures showed a fractional pattern of injury, wound healing, and dermal remodeling, while sparing the epidermis and key adnexal structures. There were zones of denatured collagen, separated by zones of spared dermis. They also discovered an increase in transforming growth factor β

(TGF-β), matrix metalloproteinases-1 and 13, and heat shock proteins 47 and 72, tropoelastin, fibrillin, as well as procollagen 1 and 3. These molecules further induced neocollagenesis and neoelastogenesis.[4] Subsequently, alternative ablative technology called "**sublative radiofrequency**" was introduced for skin resurfacing. This technology creates a low-density fractional epidermal and superficial dermal coagulation under the conductive pins and delivers RF traveling through the reticular dermis combining a low-density ablative effect in the epidermis with subnecrotic heating in deeper layers of the skin.[5]

This chapter reviews the clinical application of microneedling RF. These devices may be classified according to their type of thermal delivery pattern through the skin: sublative fractional RF, Microneedling RF with insulated needles, and Microneedling RF with non-insulated needles.

7.4 Devices and Specification

7.4.1 Sublative Fractional RF (Bipolar Fractional RF)

This type of RF uses microneedles or electrode pairs to deliver the radiofrequency energy to the skin, while the high heat at contact points creates ablation of the epidermis. Sublative RF is capable of improving superficial irregularities with minimal downtime (▶ Table 7.1).

7.4.2 Microneedle RF with Insulated Needles

The first generation of MRF systems covered most of the needle length and left only a small part of the tip non-insulated to protect the superficial epidermis, thus resulting in a small sphere-like shape coagulation zone in dermis. Multiple passes with different depths are required to cover entire dermal layers (▶ Table 7.2).

Table 7.1 Sublative fractional RF (bipolar fractional RF)

Device name	Hand piece	Unique features
Fractora (Invasix, Israel)	60 pin tip array that provides 10% surface coverage and a 20 pin tip for the lower lid, upper lid, lip lines and vascular lesions. Coated vs. noncoated pin can be chosen. The coated needles are insulated along 2,000 μm, leaving the distal 500 μm uncoated	Create ablative crater (cone-type sublative resurfacing as seen in CO_2 resurfacing) combined with deep dermal subnecrotic heating
eMatrix (Syneron-Candela, Irvine, CA)	High-density 144 pin tip or standard 64 gold-covered pin. Energy up to 25 J (60–100 mJ/pin) can be delivered to the skin directly with a 5 or 10% coverage rate, through a 200 μm diameter pin. This device can penetrate up to 450 μm in the dermis	Cause strong focal heating mainly in the mid-dermis due to specific tissue conductivity when compared with fractional resurfacing which causes extensive epidermal damage with less damage in the dermis[6]
Venus Viva (Venus Concept, Toronto, CA)	The SmartScan tip provides more than 1,000 pulses of energy, penetration depth of up to 500 μm. Nanofractional RF is delivered through 160 pin per tip, with a maximum energy of 62 mJ per 1 pin with 150 × 20 μm	Due to smaller pin size, this device is claimed to reduce side effect and recovery time. A retrospective study of 43 subjects showed an efficacy of this device for various facial dermatologic conditions such as rhytides, hyperpigmentation or redness.[7] Another study in 12 patients, there were an improvement on facial pigmentation, texture and wrinkle evaluated by baseline and posttreatment photograph and through software-assisted quantification following a single treatment[8]

Abbreviation: RF, radiofrequency.

Table 7.2 Microneedle RF with insulated needles

Device name	Hand piece	Unique features
INFINI (Lutronic, Inc., Burlington, MA)	Insulated 200-μm diameter micro-needles arranged in a 7 × 7 array (49 microneedles) with a total spot size of 10 × 10 mm and 16 needle tip (5 × 5 mm). The newer model come with large 144 12 × 12 electrodes 20 × 20 mm or small 64 8 × 8 electrodes 10 × 10 mm for sublative RF mode	Smaller needle size. Create three-dimensional coagulation zone. Spare epidermis and DEJ eliminates the need for cooling and risk of post-inflammatory hyperpigmentation. Adjust depth from 0.5 to 3.5 mm, exposure time from 10 to 1,000 ms leading to more control over tissue damage. A multicenter safety pilot study used the highest RF energies (over 100 mJ/pin) total 4 KJ per treatment demonstrated a high degree of tolerability with 1 to 2 days of downtime. By 1 week, all side effects resolved in 77% of subjects.[9]
INTRAcel (Jeisys Medical, Seoul, South Korea)	49 partially insulated microneedles per cm^2. Each electrode is 1.5 mm in length with distal 0.3 mm uninsulated emitting RF wave. The diameter of one microneedle is 100 to 200 μm. Controlled depth 0.5 to 2 mm	These microneedle electrodes emit and directly deliver RF waves at the dermal level while sparing the epidermis. Four modes of different applications: bipolar, monopolar, No RF needling and Noninvasive fractional surface modality

Abbreviations: DEJ, dermal–epidermal junction; MRF, microneedling radiofrequency; RF, radiofrequency.

The newer models have a temperature control sensor. The software is programmed to emit energy until preselected target temperatures are reached to maintain temperature for the desired duration for optimal collagen denaturation (▶ Table 7.3).

7.4.3 Microneedling RF with Non-Insulated Needles

Non-insulated needles have the ability to eliminate microbleeding during treatment due to effective coagulation and a broad electric field through the papillary and reticular dermis along the full length of the needles. Harth et al studied the histologic effect of the non-insulated microneedle RF on animal skin. Histologic examination showed clear mechanical disruption of the epidermis related to needle penetration with minimal thermal damage. The mechanical disruption closes rapidly and is nonexistent 4 days' post-therapy, a finding implying that there is less significant epidermal damage (▶ Table 7.4).[10]

7.5 Acne and Acne Scar

Acne pathophysiology is complex and arises from a dysregulation of multiple processes, including imbalance in inflammatory mediators and the microbiome with overpopulation of *Propionibacterium acnes*, dystrophic hyperkeratosis of the hair follicle, and excessive sebum production. These factors lead to rupture of the follicular wall with release of hair, lipids, keratin, and *P. acnes* into the dermis causing inflammation and activation of the classic and alternative complement pathways. Disorganized and destroyed collagen and elastic fibers from fibroblastic dysregulation around the inflamed follicle leads to the appearance of acne scar. There are three types of atrophic acne scar: ice pick, rolling scar (superficial and deep soft scar), and boxcar scar (depressed fibrotic scar). Each subtype has a varying degree of response to different treatment options. Depressed scars may reach up to 0.7 mm depth. Therefore, effective treatment will have to reach beyond this point to mechanically disrupt the dystrophic tissue.[11]

There is no standard of care for the treatment of acne scars due to the difference in type and degree of scars on every patient. Options for the reduction of acne scars include punch excision, punch grafting, surgical excision, subcision, dermabrasion, chemical peelings, injection of

Table 7.3 MRF with insulated needles and temperature control sensor

Device name	Hand piece	Unique features
Miratone (Primaeva Medical, Inc, Pleasanton, CA)	Five paired electrodes that are insulated, except for the distal tips extending from 0.75 to 2 mm beneath the skin surface. Build-in temperatures sensor	Real-time temperature feedback programmed to emit energy until preselected target temperatures are attained and to maintain temperature for a desired duration for optimal collagen denaturation
ePrime; now known as Profound (Syneron-Candela, Yokneam Illit, Israel)	Five microneedle electrode pairs deployed into the dermis at an angle of 20 to 25 degrees with the exposed portion extending from 1 to 2 mm beneath the skin surface. The proximal half of each 6-mm microneedle is electrically insulated	Intelligent Feedback System assesses the temperature of treatment site every 10th second by means of the temperature probe at the end of the needle to maintain the target temperature across a wide range of clinically relevant dermal impedance

Abbreviation: MRF, microneedling radiofrequency.

Table 7.4 MRF with non-insulated needles

Device name	Hand piece	Unique features
Intensif (EndyMed Medical, Caesarea, Israel)	25 non-insulated gold plated microneedle electrodes. The needle penetration depth was up to 3.5 mm in digitally controlled increments of 0.1 mm. The power is adjustable from 0 to 25 W. Exposure time ranges from 30 to 200 ms	Needles sharply tapered at tip. Needle depth penetration controlled by digital program with smooth motion to reduce patient discomfort. The built-in electronic board uses the electrical impedance differences between the epidermis (high impedance) and the dermis (low impedance) to further increase the dermal selectivity
Scarlet (Viol Co., Korea)	25 non-insulated microneedle electrode per the area of 10 mm², with the exposed electrode extending from 0.5 to 3 mm with 0.1 mm increment with 0.3 mm diameter	Control electrodes using advanced technology (Shock Free Needles) to minimize pain. Adjustable RF voltage up to a maximum of 40 V can be delivered, in relation to the intensity (1–10) and conduction time (100–800 m seconds)

Abbreviations: MRF, microneedling radiofrequency; RF, radiofrequency.

fillers, and a variety of laser skin resurfacing procedures such as ablative, non-ablative, and fractional laser technologies alone or best, in combination.

Ong and Bashi reviewed the use of the fractional photothermolysis (FP) for acne scar treatments including 13 ablative and 13 non-ablative FP devices. For ablative FP, the improvement ranged from 26 to 83% with facial erythema lasting 3 to 14 days and PIH in up to 92.3% of patients, whereas for non-ablative FP, efficacy varied from 26 to 50% with facial erythema for 1 to 3 days and PIH in up to 13% of patients.[12] Even though ablative FP showed superior efficacy, the incidence of PIH limits its use in darker skinned patients.

7.5.1 MRF for Acne Treatment

In 2005, Prieto et al reported 32 patients with moderate acne who were treated twice-weekly for 4 weeks with a combination of pulsed light and RF energy. The result revealed 47% reduction in mean lesion count ($p < 0.05$). The percentage of follicles with perifolliculitis decreased from 58 to 33%, and sebaceous gland areas decreased from 0.092 to 0.07 mm².

The improvement of acne might be due to reduction in some sebaceous glands and/or a reduction in perifolliculitis.[13]

Since the overproduction of sebaceous gland activity is a main pathophysiological factor in acne, Kobayashi used a 1.50-mm-long needle with a 0.45 mm base insulation inserted into pores in the forehead and cheeks, and a high-frequency electrical current was applied for 0.25 to 0.50 seconds with an output of 40 W. The mean reduction rate of skin surface lipids was 31.5% by sebumeter measurement ($p < 0.01$) at 6-month follow-up. Histology showed fewer sebaceous glands and the development of fibrosis.[14] Lee et al discovered a favorable effect of MRF **Scartlet (Viol Co., Korea)** on moderate to severe pustular acne.[11] After two treatments monthly, using intensity 7 at 3 mm depth for two passes, there was a significant improvement in acne lesion count and severity. Another study confirmed the sebosuppressive effect of MRF. Twenty Korean subjects with moderate to severe acne received a single treatment of **INFINI (Lutronic, Inc., Burlington, MA)** to the full face at energy level 5, exposure time of 50 to 100 ms at 1.0 to 1.5 mm depth.

CSL (casual sebum level) and SER (sebum excretion rate) showed 30 to 60% and 70 to 80% reduction, respectively, at week 2 ($p < 0.01$), and remained below the baseline level until week 8. Acne lesion count revealed clinical improvement with maximum efficacy at week 2 but returning to baseline in most patients by week 8. The findings imply there is long-term effect of MRF on sebaceous gland, but short-term effect for acne control after a single treatment of MRF.[15]

Kim et al[16]evaluated the efficacy of MRF using **INTRAcel (Jeisys Medical, Seoul, South Korea)** in 25 patients with moderate to severe acne. The treatment was done three times monthly with exposure time of 80 ms, power level 3, and 1.5 mm depth. The result showed statistically significant reductions in acne lesions at 4, 8, and 12 weeks after treatment compared with baseline with inflammatory lesions responding better than noninflammatory lesions. The mean decrease in sebum secretion at 1 month after the third treatment was 42.18%. Sebum secretion increased slowly subsequently but remained lower than baseline until 3 months after treatment. With multiple treatments, a more prolonged control of active acne lesions was demonstrated.

Shin et al performed a comparative split-face study to evaluate the efficacy and safety of **Fractional CO_2 laser (10,600 nm) versus MRF (Scarlet)** for active acne treatment. Fractional CO_2 was done at 80 mJ and 100 spots/cm^2 for two passes. MRF treatment setting was at intensity level 8, density of 25 MTZ/cm2 at 1.5 to 2.5 mm depth. Both showed improvement in acne with no significant differences in physician-measured parameters, patient ratings, or intraoperative pain. Downtime was significantly longer for the fractional CO_2-treated side (11.75 vs. 2.35 days). Most patients refused to do another CO_2 treatment due to the extended period of erythema. Two cases of PIH occurred only on the CO_2-treated side.[17] MRF proved to be more convenient and tolerable to most of the patients.

Postinflammatory erythema (PIE) is very common following inflammatory acne and is cosmetically unacceptable to patients. Min et al conducted a retrospective review of 25 patients treated with two sessions of **INFINI**. There was a significant difference in the degree of erythema from investigator grading, photometric measurement, and imaging analysis by software between MRF group and control group. Furthermore, histologic studies revealed reduced inflammation, microvessels, interleukin 8 (IL-8), Nuclear Factor kappa-light-chain-enhancer of activated B cells (NF-kB), and vascular endothelial growth factor (VEGF) after treatment. MRF may be an effective treatment for PIE due to anti-inflammatory and antiangiogenetic properties.[18]

7.5.2 MRF for Acne Scar Treatment

A review of six studies comprised of 121 patients compared the treatment efficacy of bipolar RF, unipolar RF, and fractional RF and demonstrated that out of all RF modalities, microneedle bipolar and fractional bipolar RF offer the best result for acne scarring. 25–75% improvement is usually achieved in 3 months posttreatment.[19]

Kaminaka et al first studied the histology from punch biopsies of acne scar patients who underwent sublative fractional RF. The results showed that sublative fractional RF with two passes caused deep thermal injury depth with denaturation of sebaceous glands and hair follicles in the dermis. The results indicated that sublative fractional RF can lead to remodeling in the deep dermal structure.[20] The same authors consequently performed a clinical study of five treatment sessions of **eMatrix (Syneron, Yokneam Illit, Israel)** on patients with acne and atrophic scar. The treatment parameter was 64 pins, peak energy was 62 mJ/pin, and coverage was 10%. They noted marked improvement in scar volume among the patients with mild scars. At least moderate improvement was achieved in 57.5% of the treated areas. The treated areas exhibited significantly fewer lesions compared with baseline at each time point ($p < 0.05$). Patient's quality of life also improved considerably. Furthermore, significant reductions in the patients' sebum levels, skin roughness, and scar depth were observed. However, 10% of subjects experienced a flare-up of acneiform lesions at the end of the study.[21]

A new generation of **eMatrix** was developed to maximize the ability to deliver energy up to 100 mJ/pin. In a Chinese study, patients received four monthly high-energy (85–95 mJ/pin) treatments with this RF device. Evaluation of global improvement and satisfaction increased at the 12 week assessment visit compared with baseline.[22] Phothong et al performed a split-face, double-blinded, randomized control trial using a high-energy setting of 100 mJ/pin versus a moderate setting of 60 mJ/pin in order to treat acne scar. The side of the face receiving higher energy demonstrated statistically significant improvement versus the moderate energy side ($p = 0.03$). Pain score and the duration of erythema after treatment were significantly higher on the high energy side as well. Also, post-inflammatory hyperpigmentation (PIH) developed 17.5% on high energy side compared to 13.3% on moderate energy side.[23]

Hellman reported a retrospective review of patients who underwent **Fractora (Invasix, Israel)** treatment. Eight patients received four treatment sessions with the initial doses of 20 to 40 mJ/pin; the doses increased each visit, based on patient tolerance. Histology specimens were collected from two patients pre- and posttreatment. All participants had a significant improvement assessed by photography. Biopsy after treatment demonstrated that scar thickness diminished in depth from 1.5 to 0.8 mm with newly formed collagen fibers, adnexal structure, and elastic tissue.[24] A subsequent follow-up study with four out of eight patients demonstrated the improvement increased over time during a follow-up period ranging from 4 months to 2 years.[25] Another prospective trial using **Intensif (EndyMed Medical, Caesarca, Israel)** for acne scar treatment revealed a global aesthetic improvement scale of excellent in 25% of patients, good in 50%, and minimal in 20%.[10]

MRF for Acne Scar Treatment in Darker Skin Type

Cho et al revealed the grade of acne scars improved in 73.3% of Korean patients after two treatment of **INTRAcel** using 1.5-mm-needle depth. Interestingly, enlarged pores also improved in 70% of participants which were confirmed by image analysis with the area of facial pores decreasing by 58.7% ($p < 0.001$). The side effects were mild including pain, erythema, and folliculitis. No PIH was observed.[26] **INTRAcel** also showed a favorable effect in Thai subjects. Twenty-six patients underwent three monthly treatment sessions using energy level 3, 30 W, exposure time 80 ms for two passes. In a group with mean scar age of

7 years (range: 0.5–15 years), all subjects (100%) rated at least 25 to 50% overall satisfaction, whereas physician graded 82% of the subject having at least 25 to 50% improvement. The risk of PIH was 3.85%. An objective evaluation using Visioscan demonstrated statistically significant improvement of skin roughness ($p = 0.012$) and scar volume ($p = 0.03$) at 1-month follow-up, but no further significant change at 3 and 6 months.[27]

In Indian subjects, Chandrashekar et al performed a retrospective photograph analysis in 31 patients of skin types III to IV with acne scar. The **INFINI** system, with energy of 25 to 40 W and needle depth of 1.5 to 3.5 mm, demonstrated efficacy for treatment of acne scar evaluated by Goodman and Baron's Global Acne scarring system. Of patients with grades 3 and 4 acne scars, 80.64% showed improvement by 2 grades and 19.35% showed improvement by 1 grade. Five patients reported PIH and two had track marks of the device probe.[28] Pudukadan further evaluated the effects of MRF for treating acne scars in darker skin type patients. Nineteen patients received three treatments with **Intensif**. The treatment parameters were 15 to 25 W, exposure time of 110 to 140 ms, and needle depth of 2.0 to 3.0 mm. Improvement of at least 1 acne scar grade was noted in 11 of 19 patients (57.9%) after 1 month and 9 of 9 patients (100%) after 3 months. The investigators also observed dyschromia improvement in 9 patients (47.4%) and hypothesized that this effect resulted from destruction of "dropped" dermal melanosome.[29]

Comparative Study for Acne Scar Treatment

INFINI was more effective for ice pick and boxcar scar compared to bipolar RF Polaris WRA (**Syneron Medical INC., Yokneam, Israel**) in a 12-week prospective single-blind, randomized clinical trial. The MRF was applied at levels 2 to 3 for 50 to 70 ms. The bipolar RF delivered fluence of 100 mJ/cm² at 100 Hz. Both modalities were done with slight overlapping in three passes. Specimens obtained for this study demonstrated increased expression of TGF-β and collagen I and decreased expression of NF-κB, IL-8 on the MRF-treated side.[30] A randomized split-face clinical study in Thai patients revealed that both fractional erbium-doped glass 1,550-nm laser **Fraxel re: store DUAL 1550/1927 (Solta Medical, Hayward, CA)** and fractional bipolar RF **eMatrix (Syneron-Candela, Irvine, CA)** significantly improved acne scar and skin texture, with no statistical difference between the two devices. The **eMatrix** parameter was Program C using 53 to 59 mJ/pin for two passes. **Fraxel re:store** treatment setting was 30 to 50 mJ/MTZ with treatment levels 4 to 5, 10 to 14% coverage for eight passes. The pain score was higher and one patient (5%) had prolonged erythema and PIH in fractional erbium-doped glass 1,550-nm-treated side. However, the duration of scab shedding was shorter after the fractional erbium-doped glass treatment.[31]

Another randomized comparative study between 1,550-nm Er:Glass fractional laser and MRF was conducted in Korea. Forty patients randomly received either 1,550-nm Er:Glass fractional laser or MRF treatment. Scar severity scores (ECCA grading scale) improved by a mean of 25.0 and 18.6% for the devices, respectively, but no significant difference occurred between the group. Boxcar and rolling scar responded significantly after treatment, whereas ice pick scar did not. Again in this study, two patients developed

PIH and acneiform eruption in the fractional laser group. Overall, the MRF group had significantly less pain, shorter downtime, and fewer side effects, leading to higher patient satisfaction.[32]

7.5.3 Combining MRF with Other Modalities for Acne Scar Treatment

Fractional bipolar RF combined with diode laser/bipolar radiofrequency (DLRF) has proven effective and safe for the treatment of acne scar. DLRF was designed to create focal coagulation and necrosis of the reticular dermis at 1.5 mm skin depth as a means of stimulating neocollagenesis, while addition of the fractional bipolar RF then produces ablation of the epidermis and papillary dermis. Diode laser bipolar radiofrequency (DLRF) setting range from 60 to 70J/cm^2 with RF at 80 to 100 J/cm.[3] Then, fractional bipolar RF follows with energy 19 and 25 J (Program C, 5% coverage). With this protocol, Peterson revealed that acne scar scores statistically significantly decreased by 72.3% ($p < 0.001$), skin texture enhanced by 66.7% ($p < 0.001$) and acne scar pigmentation improved by 13.3% ($p = 0.05$) after five monthly sessions. No subjects displayed PIH.[33] Taub and Garretson found similar results. The median scar assessment scores significantly improved after three treatments out of five and persisted throughout the study. Skin type did not affect the outcome, and PIH occurred in a single patient with skin type IV but resolved without intervention.[34]

MRF has also improved a variety of acne scars while sublative RF has been shown to induce upper epidermal ablation with a column of dermal remodeling. Combining two different modalities demonstrates good results. Twenty Asian subjects with skin types III to IV received three treatments of **dual mode INFINI** monthly. MRF treatment parameter was: level 7, 50 ms, at 1.5 mm depth. Next, sublative RF was applied with treatment level 16 to 17 and 70 to 80 ms exposure time. Blinded physician assessors rated all subjects as having grade 2 or more clinical improvement; 4 (20%) had grade 4, 10 (50%) had grade 3, and 6 (30%) had grade 2 improvement. Furthermore, there was significant improvement in all three types of scar ($p < 0.05$). However, with a combination of two treatment modalities, two patients developed transient PIH, two flushing, and one worsening active acne.[35]

Subcision is a conventional method used to mechanically disrupt the fibrotic tissue in the dermis that tethers down scars. Faghihi et al conducted a randomized split-face study to evaluate the treatment efficacy of MRF (INFINI) with and without subcision. Combined treatment with subcision had a significantly better improvement graded by the two blinded dermatologists and by patient rating using a visual analog scale.[36] From our experiences, combining MRF with subcision showed beneficial results with minimal risk of downtime and adverse effects (▶ Fig. 7.1).

7.6 Rejuvenation

One histologic hallmark of photodamaged skin is the accumulation of elastin-containing fibrils in the papillary dermis and mid-dermis, known as solar elastosis. Collagen fibers also become disorganized and breakdown. These changes manifest clinically as fine lines, rhytides, dyschromia, telangiectasia, and skin laxity. Reversal of these changes can be achieved via the selective application of energy devices including lasers, lights, ultrasound, and radiofrequency.

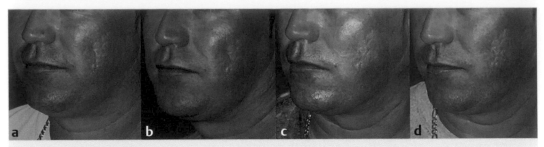

Fig. 7.1 A 30-year-old man with scattered rolling, pitted, boxcar acne scars—more prominent left side. **(a)** The baseline photo, **(b)** 1 month, **(c)** 2 months and **(d)** 3 months follow-up after monthly treatment with Microneedling RF (INFINI) combined with subcision showed a moderate degree of improvement.

7.6.1 MRF for Facial Rejuvenation

Sublative fractional RF creates an ablative epidermal injury plus deep dermal coagulative damage. In a multicenter trial, 20 Caucasian (skin types I and II) and 30 Asian patients (skin types III and IV) received a single full-face, ablative fractional radiofrequency treatment using the **Fractora** hand piece. The investigators used energy of 50 to 62 mJ/pin for light skin and 10 to 40 mJ/pin for darker skin. Histologic samples were taken immediately after treatment and at 1, 2, and 6 weeks posttreatment to analyze the character of fractional lesions and the wound healing process. With a high setting of 60 mJ/pin, the ablation crater depth reached 500 to 600 µm, going through the epidermis, the papillary dermis to mid-deep reticular dermis. The architecture and shape of the zone of ablation was a typical "cone-shaped" lesion, similar to that seen with CO_2 ablative lasers. The zone of coagulation measured at 60 to 100 µm surrounding the ablation crater. The improvement of Asian versus Caucasian skin texture was 70 versus 67%; pores was 40 versus 22%; wrinkles and lines were 45 versus 63%; acne scars were 40 versus 40%; and pigmentation was 30 versus 60%, respectively.[37] Another study revealed the efficacy and safety of sublative fractional RF for facial rejuvenation. A single-center, prospective study enrolled 25 female subjects between the ages of 35 to 60 years. Each subject underwent three full-face treatments using **eMatrix** at monthly intervals. All treatments were delivered with energy between 40 to 50 mJ. At 6 months following the final RF treatment, photodamage, skin laxity, texture, fine lines, and wrinkles were analyzed. There was a statistically significant difference noted in appearance of the Fitzpatrick–Goldman wrinkle scale between the baseline and posttreatment photographs ($p < 0.001$).[38]

A multicenter study of the efficacy and safety for treatment of facial wrinkles using the **INFINI** system included 499 patients with Fitzpatrick skin types I to V from five study centers in Italy, India, Korea, Poland, and Turkey. They used a large variety of treatment parameters employed across multiple centers. Needle depth ranged from 0.5 to 3 mm, power level from 4 to 12, and exposure time from 20 to 200 ms through one to three passes. Clinical improvement evaluated by dermatologists and patient satisfaction as a 5-part scale showed a similar result of over 80% average improvement. Side effects were mild with PIH seen in five patients (2.3%) from the Italian center.[39] In our experience, MRF is a useful device for improving skin texture of certain cosmetic area such as perioral rhytids.

The step-by-step treatment procedure is illustrated in ▶ Fig. 7.2a–f.

The application of MRF to Asian skin types has also been studied. Twenty-five women (mean age 54.2; Fitzpatrick skin phototypes III–IV) received three consecutive fractional RF treatments (**Scarlet**) at 4-week intervals with nonoverlap passes. Results included improvement in hydration and skin roughness ($p < 0.05$). Histologic examination revealed marked increase in dermal thickness, dermal collagen, and fibrillin content.[40] The same investigators further showed the synergistic effect of human stem cell conditioned medium on fractional RF treatment using

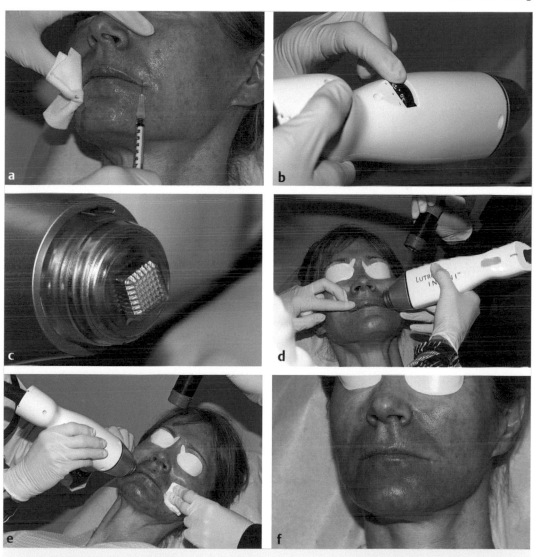

Fig. 7.2 A step-by-step figure of the treatment process. A 56-year-old female patient presented for perioral rhytides treatment. **(a)** For pain control, patient was pretreated with topical or inject anesthetic agent. **(b)** The energy setting and the depth of treatment depends on patient condition. The figure shows the adjustable depth of the needles. **(c)** Insulated 200-μm-diameter microneedle arranged in a 7 × 7 array (49 microneedles) **(d)** The handpiece optimally contacts with the skin during the treatment process. Simultaneously, Zimmer air cooler helps for cooling the epidermis **(e)** Pinpoint bleeding is commonly observed with this type of insulated needles. **(f)** Immediately posttreatment, the patient had mild degree of erythema, which resolved in a few days. (Images courtesy of Dr. Kimberly Butterwick.)

a randomized, controlled split-face study. They found evidence of proteins from the human stem cell conditioned medium in both the epidermis and the dermis after treatment.[41]

7.6.2 MRF for Lower Face and Neck Laxity

Treatment of neck skin needs to take into account the unique anatomical features of this region including generally thinner skin, greater laxity, and fewer pilosebaceous units resulting in slower healing and a necessity for increased caution. Fractional ablative laser can be used judiciously in this area, though results tend to be modest.[42] Non-ablative laser is useful for the treatment of dyschromia and wrinkles but not effective for skin laxity.[43] MRF has proven to be both safe and effective in the treatment of neck skin laxity.

In a prospective multicenter clinical trial using **ePrime, Syneron-Candela, Yokneam Illit, Israel** (**Profound**), 100 subjects with mild to severe facial and neck rhytides and laxity (mean age: 54.5) received one single-pass treatment at a preselected real-time fixed temperature of 62 to 78 °C, energy duration for 3 to 5 seconds, impedance restrictions of 200 to 3,000 Ohms. Participants obtained a mean improvement of 25.6% on the Fitzpatrick–Goldman wrinkle scale and 24.1% on the Alexiades–Armenakas laxity scale at 6 months. However, superficial needle insertion caused two incidences of punctate atrophy.[44]

Additionally, the efficacy of MRF was confirmed by an international multicenter study in the United States and Japan.[45] Forty-nine patients completed three monthly treatments using **Intensif**. The cheek area received treatment with exposure time of 110 to 140 ms, power of 10 to 20 W, and depth of 1.8 to 2.8 mm. The neck area received treatment with exposure time of 80 to 140 ms, power of 10 to 20 W, and depth of 1.3 to 2.5 mm. Improvement in Fitzpatrick–Goldman wrinkle and elastosis scale was seen in 100% of the patients. Sixty-five percent of patients had significant improvement. In another study using computer measurements of improvement in gnathion and cervicomental angles, 35 patients received three monthly treatments with **INFINI**. There was a significant posttreatment decrease in gnathion and cervicomental angles of 28.5 and 16.6 degrees, respectively, at 6-month follow-up. A "telephone survey" at 1 year after the treatment implied lasting satisfaction.[46]

A randomized, blinded study compared 15 patients who underwent a single treatment of MRF **Miratone** (**Primaeva Medical, Inc, Pleasanton, California**) with six surgical facelift patients. In the MRF group, subjects received treatment at 62 to 78 °C for 3 to 5 seconds. Those patients in MRF group achieved a mean grade correction of 0.44 on a 4-point laxity grading scale, whereas facelift patients improved 1.20 ($p < 0.001$). The improvements relative to baseline were 16% for MRF treatment compared with 49% for surgery, or a single MRF treatment yielded results equivalent to 37% that of the facelift. Based on these findings, the authors concluded that MRF treatment might provide an important nonsurgical option for the treatment of facial skin laxity.[47]

7.6.3 MRF for Treatment Periorbital Wrinkles

Repetitive muscle contractions plus cumulative ultraviolet-induced photoaging give rise to periorbital wrinkling. MRF has been successfully used to achieve rejuvenation of this area. In a Korean study, 11 women with skin type III to IV and a mean Fitzpatrick–Goldman wrinkle classification system scoring at 5.59 unit completed three sessions of MRF treatment using **RFXEL (Medipark, Uiwang-si, Gyeonggi-do, Korea)**. The energy level was 20 with pulse duration of 0.4 second at 2 mm depth for two passes. At 3-month follow-up, they found significant improvement ($p < 0.001$) with a mean reduction in Fitzpatrick wrinkle classification system scoring at 2.2 unit. PIH was not observed.[48] Another prospective study included 20 Korean patients with Fitzpatrick skin type IV to V. All subjects were treated using bipolar mode of **INTRAcel** three times at 4-week intervals (0.8 mm depth, power 12.5, 100 ms). Follow-up results at 6 months showed statistically significant improvement of mean 5-point wrinkle assessment scale ($p < 0.001$)[49] In this study, two patients reported mild PIH, which resolved within 4 weeks.

Compared to intradermal botulinum toxin type A (BoNT-A), BoNT-A injection was superior to MRF at short-term follow-up but inferior at long-term follow-up. BoNT-A was more efficacious 3 weeks after treatment. However, MRF (**INFINI**), performed at a depth of 0.5 mm for 80 ms with 150 W (level 6) intensity for two passes at 0, 3, and 6 weeks showed improvement at 18 weeks. Skin biopsies found increased expression of procollagen-3 and elastin on the MRF side compared to the untreated skin and the BoNT-A injection side. These results imply that MRF therapy produce gradual and long-term benefits in periorbital rejuvenation.[50]

7.6.4 MRF for Treatment Nasal and Perioral Wrinkles

Some patients complain of age-related change of nose such as drooping nasal tip secondary to underlying bone atrophy. **Intensif** showed preliminary effects on nonsurgical tightening and shaping of nasal tip as well as rejuvenation of perioral area shown in three-dimensional imaging study in 15 Asian patients Fitzpatrick skin type III to IV after a single treatment. The procedure parameters were 80 to 110 ms at 12 to 14 W and 1.5 to 2.5 mm depth.[51]

7.7 MRF for Other Conditions

7.7.1 MRF for Axillary Hyperhidrosis Treatment

Primary axillary hyperhidrosis (PAH) involves excessive sweat production due to malfunction of the autonomic nervous system. Although there are several conservative treatment options including aluminum chloride, tap water iontophoresis, anticholinergic drugs, or BoNT, results of these modalities are temporary with neuromodulator effects on sweat gland production lasting 6 to 18 months, depending on the dosage utilized. Surgical treatment by curettage and/or skin excision typically has an undesirable side effect profile of postoperative delayed healing, pain, and scarring. Sympathetic nerve block has the adverse effect of producing compensatory sweating elsewhere.

Denaturation of proteins at high temperature, resulting in permanent damage to the sweat gland, is the likely mechanism for MRF in the treatment of hyperhidrosis. Kim et al[52] introduced the use of MRF for PAH in a pilot study. Based on the report that microwave devices had long-term effects on the treatment of PAH causing irreversible thermolysis of the apocrine and eccrine sweat gland,[53] 20 Asian patients with hyperhidrosis disease severity scale (HDSS) grade 3 to 4 received two treatments at monthly interval with **INFINI**. They took into account the fact that sweat glands arise at an average skin depth of 3.5 mm of skin[54] when designing their protocol, and histology confirmed coagulative necrosis immediately after treatment. HDSS significantly improve after treatment. 75% and 60% of the patients reached an HDSS score of 1 or 2 after 4 and 8 weeks of follow-up, respectively. By comparison, a study using BoNT found that 85 and 90% of patients reached HDSS score of 1 or 2 after 4 and 12 weeks of follow-up.[55] Although the result of MRF was slightly less efficient, it permanently destroyed apocrine and eccrine glands versus the temporary effects of BoNT-A. In this study, no subjects experienced major side effects. Two patients developed compensatory hyperhidrosis in other areas of the body. One complained of transient numbness of her right arm. Another controlled study demonstrated that the HDSS and VAS significantly improved on the treated side in comparison to control. Follow-up evaluation revealed that 79% of the patients had a 1- or 2-point decrease in HDSS.[56]

Schick et al revealed the efficacy of MRF for a treatment of axillary hyperhidrosis in 30 patients with grade 3 to 4 of HDSS. The average subjective reduction of sweating was 72%, and HDSS scores and DLQI improved significantly after three treatment sessions at 6-week intervals ($p < 0.05$). Objective quantitative measurement using gravimetry also revealed a statistically significant reduction in sweat from 221 mg/min at baseline to 33 mg/min ($p < 0.05$), a final level which is just slightly above the normal sweating of 30 mg/minute. Side effects included exudation or scab (87%), irregular growth of axillary hair (56%), arm twitching during the procedure (27%), mildly reduced sensitivity (20%), and superficial ulceration (7%). PIH was not observed in this study.[57]

Treatment of PAH with MRF is a promising noninvasive option with good therapeutic effects and few, if any, long-lasting side effects. Further studies should be performed to establish the most beneficial treatment protocol.

7.7.2 MRF for Rosacea Treatment

The hypothesis that MRF may treat rosacea came from data in management of inflammatory acne[15,16,58] and acne-related post inflammatory erythema.[18] A prospective, randomized, split-face, clinical trial investigated the clinical and histological impact of **MRF (INFINI)** among rosacea patients. Park et al demonstrated a modest but statistically significant improvement on the treated side, evaluated by clinical rating and photometric measurement, after two monthly treatment sessions. Histological and immunological sampling showed a reduction of inflammatory cell count, mast cell, VEGF, NF-κB and IL-8, LL-37, and TLR-2 and transient receptor potential vanilloid (TRPV-2, TRPV-3, TRPV-4) compared with baseline. At week 12, patients reported improvement in papules or pustules (57.5%), persistent erythema (28.2%), burning sensation (27.9%), and transient erythema (25.6%). Interestingly, MRF was slightly more efficient in reducing erythema in patients with papulopustular than erythematotelangiectatic subtypes. Correlated with these histological results, MRF may have an anti-inflammatory and antiangiogenesis effect. Further studies should confirm the efficacy of this device in rosacea patients.[59]

7.7.3 MRF for Striae Distensae Treatment

Striae distensae (SD) are common yet cosmetically unacceptable to many patients.

In early stages, SD are pink or red (striae rubra) and gradually develop atrophic changes, resulting in white wrinkling (striae alba). Several factors are responsible for striae formation: genetics, obesity, rapid linear growth, mechanical stress from pregnancy, and topical or systemic corticosteroids. Currently, there is no universally successful or optimal therapeutic choice. Fractional photothermolysis or pulsed dye laser are recommended treatments for SD, but results are unpredictable.[60,61,62]

The mechanism of MRF in SD treatment may relate to dermal remodeling and growth factor stimulation from bulk heating of the dermis. In 2013, Ryu et al conducted a study to evaluate the effect of MRF combination with fractional CO_2 laser. Thirty Korean patients with Fitzpatrick skin type IV were randomized to receive MRF only, CO_2 only, or both. After three monthly treatments, the combination group showed greater clinical improvement based on ratings from two blinded dermatologists and patients. Mean clinical improvement score was 1.8 in the MRF-treated group, 2.2 in the fractional CO_2 laser-treated group, and 3.4 in the combination group. Skin biopsy after combination treatment revealed epidermal thickening, increased numbers of collagen bundles, and high expression of TGF-β1. Interestingly, there was also increased quantity of stratifin, a novel keratinocyte-derived protein molecule, which has a crucial role in keratinocyte differentiation, intracellular functions, regulation of signal transduction pathways, cellular trafficking, as well as cell proliferation and differentiation.[63] Greater expression of TGF-β1 and stratifin is likely responsible for accumulation and thickening of the collagen fibers in the dermis. Transient PIH occurred in all groups but most commonly after combination therapy.[64]

Later, Fatemi Naeini et al performed another comparative study showing the efficacy in Iranian patients. Forty-eight pairs of striae alba from six patients were randomized to left and right sides receiving treatment either with MRF (**INFINI**) alone or MRF with fractional CO_2 laser. The mean difference of the surface area between pre- and posttreatment in the combination group was significantly higher than that in the MFR only group ($p = 0.003$). Clinical improvement scales showed significantly better response in the combination than MRF group at the first and second follow up ($p = 0.002$ and 0.004). Intraoperative pain was similar between both groups. However, transient PIH was observed significantly more often in the combination group ($p = 0.004$).[65] Both of the described studies show that MRF in conjunction with fractional CO_2 laser may be promising options in the treatment of striae distensae without serious side effect.

A nanofractional radiofrequency device **Venus Viva (Venus Concept, Toronto, CA)** has also been applied to the treatment of SD. Thirty-three Thai subjects enrolled for a total of three sessions at 4-week intervals. At 1 month after treatment, the total area (the width and the length) of striae alba significantly decreased from that at baseline ($p < 0.001$). Pathology found significantly increased number of collagen and elastin bundles. Eighteen percent of patients reported transient PIH.[66] Compared to PIH occurring after treatment of striae alba with fractional CO_2 laser (81.8%) or Erbium glass laser (36.4%),[67] the rate from MRF is relatively low.

In summary, MRF as well as ablative and non-ablative lasers all have a role in treating SD with the choice of treatment dependent on the skin type of the patient. Regardless of modality, multiple treatment sessions are essential to achieve optimal results. We also suggest that the addition of topical growth factors immediately after treatment may further potentiate the efficacy and continued topical application may enhance fibroblastic function.

7.8 Side Effects

Skin types III to VI tend to have an increased risk of PIH following exposure to laser or energy-based devices. Although a laser-based FP system significantly lowers the risk of adverse events compared with conventional nonfractionated laser skin resurfacing, PIH can still occur in up to 40% of non-ablative and 92% of ablative FP treatments.[68] Adverse events of MRF are limited to mild pain, transient erythema or edema, and rarely epidermal atrophy after the procedure. Fewer patients demonstrate PIH.[39,49] Skin depressions have been reported and is thought to be due to superficial placement of the hand piece, using too high energy at the upper level of the skin, or uneven facial contours.[44]

References

[1] Mutalik S. Radiofrequency in dermatosurgery. J Cutan Aesthet Surg. 2008; 1(2):94
[2] Baris R, Kankaya Y, Ozer K, et al. The effect of microneedling with a roller device on the viability of random skin flaps in rats. Plast Reconstr Surg. 2013; 131(5):1024–1034
[3] Fernandes D. Minimally invasive percutaneous collagen induction. Oral Maxillofac Surg Clin North Am. 2005; 17(1):51–63, vi
[4] Hantash BM, Ubeid AA, Chang H, Kafi R, Renton B. Bipolar fractional radiofrequency treatment induces neoelastogenesis and neocollagenesis. Lasers Surg Med. 2009; 41(1):1–9
[5] Hruza G, Taub AF, Collier SL, Mulholland SR. Skin rejuvenation and wrinkle reduction using a fractional radiofrequency system. J Drugs Dermatol. 2009; 8(3):259–265
[6] Brightman L, Goldman MP, Taub AF. Sublative rejuvenation: experience with a new fractional radiofrequency system for skin rejuvenation and repair. J Drugs Dermatol. 2009; 8(11) Suppl:s9–s13
[7] Ray M, Gold M. A retrospective study of patient satisfaction following a trial of nano-fractional RF treatment. J Drugs Dermatol. 2015; 14(11):1268–1271
[8] Hongcharu W, Gold M. Expanding the clinical application of fractional radiofrequency treatment: findings on rhytides, hyperpigmentation, rosacea, and acne redness. J Drugs Dermatol. 2015; 14(11):1298–1304
[9] Cohen JL, Weiner SF, Pozner JN, et al. Multi-center pilot study to evaluate the safety profile of high energy fractionated radiofrequency with insulated microneedles to multiple levels of the dermis. J Drugs Dermatol. 2016; 15(11):1308–1312
[10] Harth Y, Elman M, Ackerman E, Frank I. Depressed acne scars—effective, minimal downtime treatment with a novel smooth motion non-insulated microneedle radiofrequency technology. Journal of Cosmetics, Dermatological Sciences and Applications. 2014; 4:212–218
[11] Zheng Z, Goo B, Kim D-Y, Kang J-S, Cho SB. Histometric analysis of skin-radiofrequency interaction using a fractionated microneedle delivery system. Dermatol Surg. 2014; 40(2):134–141
[12] Ong MWS, Bashir SJ. Fractional laser resurfacing for acne scars: a review. Br J Dermatol. 2012; 166(6):1160–1169
[13] Prieto VG, Zhang PS, Sadick NS. Evaluation of pulsed light and radiofrequency combined for the treatment of acne vulgaris with histologic analysis of facial skin biopsies. J Cosmet Laser Ther. 2005; 7(2):63–68
[14] Kobayashi T, Tamada S. Selective electrothermolysis of the sebaceous glands: treatment of facial seborrhea. Dermatol Surg. 2007; 33(2):169–177
[15] Lee KR, Lee EG, Lee HJ, Yoon MS. Assessment of treatment efficacy and sebosuppressive effect of fractional radiofrequency microneedle on acne vulgaris. Lasers Surg Med. 2013; 45(10):639–647
[16] Kim ST, Lee KH, Sim HJ, Suh KS, Jang MS. Treatment of acne vulgaris with fractional radiofrequency microneedling. J Dermatol. 2014; 41(7):586–591
[17] Shin JU, Lee SH, Jung JY, Lee JH. A split-face comparison of a fractional microneedle radiofrequency device and fractional carbon dioxide laser therapy in acne patients. J Cosmet Laser Ther. 2012; 14(5):212–217
[18] Min S, Park SY, Yoon JY, Kwon HH, Suh DH. Fractional microneedling radiofrequency treatment for acne-related post-inflammatory erythema. Acta Derm Venereol. 2016; 96(1):87–91
[19] Simmons BJ, Griffith RD, Falto-Aizpurua LA, Nouri K. Use of radiofrequency in cosmetic dermatology: focus on nonablative treatment of acne scars. Clin Cosmet Investig Dermatol. 2014; 7:335–339
[20] Kaminaka C, Uede M, Nakamura Y, Furukawa F, Yamamoto Y. Histological studies of facial acne and atrophic acne scars treated with a bipolar fractional radiofrequency system. J Dermatol. 2014; 41(5):435–438
[21] Kaminaka C, Uede M, Matsunaka H, Furukawa F, Yamamoto Y. Clinical studies of the treatment of facial atrophic acne scars and acne with a bipolar fractional radiofrequency system. J Dermatol. 2015; 42(6):580–587
[22] Qin X, Li H, Jian X, Yu B. Evaluation of the efficacy and safety of fractional bipolar radiofrequency with high-energy strategy for treatment of acne scars in Chinese. J Cosmet Laser Ther. 2015; 17(5):237–245
[23] Phothong W, Wanitphakdeedecha R, Sathaworawong A, Manuskiatti W. High versus moderate energy use of bipolar fractional radiofrequency in the treatment of acne scars: a

split-face double-blinded randomized control trial pilot study. Lasers Med Sci. 2016; 31(2):229–234

[24] Hellman J. Retrospective Study of the Use of a Fractional Radio Frequency Ablative Device in the Treatment of Acne Vulgaris and Related Acne Scars. JCDSA. 2015; 05(4):311–316

[25] Hellman J. Long term follow-up results of a fractional radio frequency ablative treatment of acne vulgaris and related acne scars. Journal of Cosmetics Dermatological Sciences and Applications. 2016; 6(3):100

[26] Cho SI, Chung BY, Choi MG, et al. Evaluation of the clinical efficacy of fractional radiofrequency microneedle treatment in acne scars and large facial pores. Dermatol Surg. 2012; 38(7 Pt 1):1017–1024

[27] Vejjabhinanta V, Wanitphakdeedecha R, Limtanyakul P, Manuskiatti W. The efficacy in treatment of facial atrophic acne scars in Asians with a fractional radiofrequency microneedle system. J Eur Acad Dermatol Venereol. 2014; 28(9): 1219–1225

[28] Chandrashekar BS, Sriram R, Mysore R, Bhaskar S, Shetty A. Evaluation of microneedling fractional radiofrequency device for treatment of acne scars. J Cutan Aesthet Surg. 2014; 7(2): 93–97

[29] Pudukadan D. Treatment of acne scars on darker skin types using a noninsulated smooth motion, electronically controlled radiofrequency microneedles treatment system. Dermatol Surg. 2017; 43 Suppl 1:S64–S69

[30] Min S, Park SY, Yoon JY, Suh DH. Comparison of fractional microneedling radiofrequency and bipolar radiofrequency on acne and acne scar and investigation of mechanism: comparative randomized controlled clinical trial. Arch Dermatol Res. 2015; 307(10):897–904

[31] Rongsaard N, Rummaneethorn P. Comparison of a fractional bipolar radiofrequency device and a fractional erbium-doped glass 1,550-nm device for the treatment of atrophic acne scars: a randomized split-face clinical study. Dermatol Surg. 2014; 40(1):14–21

[32] Chae WS, Seong JY, Jung HN, et al. Comparative study on efficacy and safety of 1550 nm Er:Glass fractional laser and fractional radiofrequency microneedle device for facial atrophic acne scar. J Cosmet Dermatol. 2015; 14(2):100–106

[33] Peterson JD, Palm MD, Kiripolsky MG, Guiha IC, Goldman MP. Evaluation of the effect of fractional laser with radiofrequency and fractionated radiofrequency on the improvement of acne scars. Dermatol Surg. 2011; 37(9):1260–1267

[34] Taub AF, Garretson CB. Treatment of acne scars of skin types II to V by Sublative fractional bipolar radiofrequency and bipolar radiofrequency combined with diode laser. J Clin Aesthet Dermatol. 2011; 4(10):18–27

[35] Park JY, Lee EG, Yoon MS, Lee IJ. The efficacy and safety of combined microneedle fractional radiofrequency and sublative fractional radiofrequency for acne scars in Asian skin. J Cosmet Dermatol. 2016; 15(2):102–107

[36] Faghihi G, Poostiyan N, Asilian A, et al. Efficacy of fractionated microneedle radiofrequency with and without adding subcision for the treatment of atrophic facial acne scars: a randomized split-face clinical study. J Cosmet Dermatol. 2017; 16(2):223–229

[37] Mulholland RS, Ahn DH, Kreindel M, Paul M. Fractional ablative radio-frequency resurfacing in Asian and Caucasian skin: a novel method for deep radiofrequency fractional skin rejuvenation. Journal of Cosmetics Dermatological Sciences and Applications. 2012; 2(3):144

[38] Bloom BS, Emer J, Goldberg DJ. Assessment of safety and efficacy of a bipolar fractionated radiofrequency device in the

treatment of photodamaged skin. J Cosmet Laser Ther. 2012; 14(5):208–211

[39] Calderhead RG, et al. The clinical efficacy and safety of microneedling fractional radiofrequency in the treatment of facial wrinkles: a multicenter study with the Infini System in 499 patients. White paper, Lutronic Corp, Goyang, South Korea (2013)

[40] Seo KY, Yoon MS, Kim DH, Lee HJ. Skin rejuvenation by microneedle fractional radiofrequency treatment in Asian skin; clinical and histological analysis. Lasers Surg Med. 2012; 44(8):631–636

[41] Seo KY, Kim DH, Lee SE, Yoon MS, Lee HJ. Skin rejuvenation by microneedle fractional radiofrequency and a human stem cell conditioned medium in Asian skin: a randomized controlled investigator blinded split-face study. J Cosmet Laser Ther. 2013; 15(1):25–33

[42] Tierney EP, Hanke CW. Ablative fractionated CO2, laser resurfacing for the neck: prospective study and review of the literature. J Drugs Dermatol. 2009; 8(8):723–731

[43] Bencini PL, Tourlaki A, Galimberti M, Pellacani G. Non-ablative fractionated laser skin resurfacing for the treatment of aged neck skin. J Dermatolog Treat. 2015; 26(3):252–256

[44] Alexiades-Armenakas M, Newman J, Willey A, et al. Prospective multicenter clinical trial of a minimally invasive temperature-controlled bipolar fractional radiofrequency system for rhytid and laxity treatment. Dermatol Surg. 2013; 39(2): 263–273

[45] Gold M, Taylor M, Rothaus K, Tanaka Y. Non-insulated smooth motion, micro-needles RF fractional treatment for wrinkle reduction and lifting of the lower face: International study. Lasers Surg Med. 2016; 48(8):727–733

[46] Clementoni MT, Munavalli GS. Fractional high intensity focused radiofrequency in the treatment of mild to Moderate laxity of the lower face and neck: a pilot study. Lasers Surg Med. 2016; 48(5):461–470

[47] Alexiades-Armenakas M, Rosenberg D, Renton B, Dover J, Arndt K. Blinded, randomized, quantitative grading comparison of minimally invasive, fractional radiofrequency and surgical face-lift to treat skin laxity. Arch Dermatol. 2010; 146 (4):396–405

[48] Kim JK, Roh MR, Park GH, Kim YJ, Jeon IK, Chang SE. Fractionated microneedle radiofrequency for the treatment of periorbital wrinkles. J Dermatol. 2013; 40(3):172–176

[49] Lee SJ, Kim J-I, Yang YJ, Nam JH, Kim W-S. Treatment of periorbital wrinkles with a novel fractional radiofrequency microneedle system in dark-skinned patients. Dermatol Surg. 2015; 41(5):615–622

[50] Jeon IK, Chang SE, Park G-H, Roh MR. Comparison of microneedle fractional radiofrequency therapy with intradermal botulinum toxin a injection for periorbital rejuvenation. Dermatology. 2013; 227(4):367–372

[51] Tanaka Y. Long-term nasal and peri-oral tightening by a single fractional noninsulated microneedle radiofrequency treatment. J Clin Aesthet Dermatol. 2017; 10(2):45–51

[52] Kim M, Shin JY, Lee J, Kim JY, Oh SH. Efficacy of fractional microneedle radiofrequency device in the treatment of primary axillary hyperhidrosis: a pilot study. Dermatology. 2013; 227(3):243–249

[53] Hong HC, Lupin M, O'Shaughnessy KF. Clinical evaluation of a microwave device for treating axillary hyperhidrosis. Dermatol Surg. 2012; 38(5):728–735

[54] Grice K, Sattar H, Baker H. The effect of ambient humidity on transepidermal water loss. J Invest Dermatol. 1972; 58(6): 343–346

[55] Solish N, Benohanian A, Kowalski JW, Canadian Dermatology Study Group on Health-Related Quality of Life in Primary Axillary Hyperhidrosis. Prospective open-label study of botulinum toxin type A in patients with axillary hyperhidrosis: effects on functional impairment and quality of life. Dermatol Surg. 2005; 31(4):405–413

[56] Fatemi Naeini F, Abtahi-Naeini B, Pourazizi M, Nilforoushzadeh MA, Mirmohammadkhani M. Fractionated microneedle radiofrequency for treatment of primary axillary hyperhidrosis: a sham control study. Australas J Dermatol. 2015; 56(4):279–284

[57] Schick CH, Grallath T, Schick KS, Hashmonai M. Radiofrequency thermotherapy for treating axillary hyperhidrosis. Dermatol Surg. 2016; 42(5):624–630

[58] Lee SJ, Goo JW, Shin J, et al. Use of fractionated microneedle radiofrequency for the treatment of inflammatory acne vulgaris in 18 Korean patients. Dermatol Surg. 2012; 38(3):400–405

[59] Park SY, Kwon HH, Yoon JY, Min S, Suh DH. Clinical and histologic effects of fractional microneedling radiofrequency treatment on rosacea. Dermatol Surg. 2016; 42(12):1362–1369

[60] Suh D-H, Chang KY, Son HC, Ryu JH, Lee SJ, Song KY. Radiofrequency and 585-nm pulsed dye laser treatment of striae distensae: a report of 37 Asian patients. Dermatol Surg. 2007; 33(1):29–34

[61] Naeini FF, Nikyar Z, Mokhtari F, Bahrami A. Comparison of the fractional CO2 laser and the combined use of a pulsed dye laser with fractional CO2 laser in striae alba treatment. Adv Biomed Res. 2014; 3:184

[62] Bak H, Kim BJ, Lee WJ, et al. Treatment of striae distensae with fractional photothermolysis. Dermatol Surg. 2009; 35 (8):1215–1220

[63] Medina A, Ghaffari A, Kilani RT, Ghahary A. The role of stratifin in fibroblast-keratinocyte interaction. Mol Cell Biochem. 2007; 305(1–2):255–264

[64] Ryu H-W, Kim SA, Jung HR, Ryoo YW, Lee KS, Cho JW. Clinical improvement of striae distensae in Korean patients using a combination of fractionated microneedle radiofrequency and fractional carbon dioxide laser. Dermatol Surg. 2013; 39(10):1452–1458

[65] Fatemi Naeini F, Behfar S, Abtahi-Naeini B, Keyvan S, Pourazizi M. Promising option for treatment of striae alba: fractionated microneedle radiofrequency in combination with fractional carbon dioxide laser. Dermatol Res Pract. 2016; 2016:2896345

[66] Pongsrihadulchai N, Chalermchai T, Ophaswongse S, Pongsawat S, Udompataikul M. An efficacy and safety of nanofractional radiofrequency for the treatment of striae alba. J Cosmet Dermatol. 2017; 16(1):84–90

[67] Yang YJ, Lee G-Y. Treatment of striae distensae with nonablative fractional laser versus ablative CO(2) fractional laser: a randomized controlled trial. Ann Dermatol. 2011; 23(4):481–489

[68] Lee HS, Lee DH, Won CH, et al. Fractional rejuvenation using a novel bipolar radiofrequency system in Asian skin. Dermatol Surg. 2011; 37(11):1611–1619

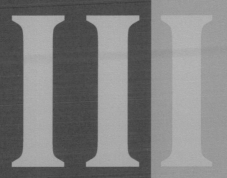

Part III

Other Considerations, Combinations, and Complications

III

8

Applications and Safety in Skin of Color

DiAnne S. Davis and Naissan O. Wesley

Abstract

As a result of increased demands for less aggressive but effective cosmetic procedures, microneedling and platelet-rich plasma (PRP) either in isolation or together have become increasingly popular treatment modalities in recent years. Enhancing one's appearance through either skin rejuvenation or the treatment of scars, striae, acne scars, pigmentary disorders (including melasma and periorbital melanosis), and even hair loss are all cosmetic concerns among a diverse patient population. While many of the listed medical conditions are amenable to ablative and/or non-ablative laser therapies, the risk of adverse events are higher among patients with skin of color, due to differences in melanocyte distribution and activity, skin reactivity, and a host of other factors; thus, there is a demand for safer yet still effective and scientifically backed therapeutic options. Microneedling and/or PRP may be just that given the lower potential for postinflammatory hyperpigmentation and scarring when compared to laser-based therapies. Both microneedling and PRP have been shown to be safe procedures on all ethnic skin types, with only minor disruption to melanocyte properties, lower risk of side effects, and a fast recovery time. In this chapter, we review current literature and offer treatment and safety recommendations for these modalities in skin of color.

Keywords: microneedling, platelet-rich plasma (PRP), skin of color, ethnic skin

Key Points

- There is an increased demand for safer procedure-based therapeutic options for many diagnoses among patients with skin of color, due to differences in melanocyte distribution, melanocyte activity, and skin reactivity.
- Microneedling and platelet-rich plasma (PRP) have been shown to be safe procedures on all ethnic skin types, with only a predisposition of keloid formation or active infections as relative contraindications.
- Microneedling may be used safely and effectively for facial rejuvenation, acne scarring, melasma, periorbital melanosis, and striae. Enhanced absorption of topical therapies may also occur after microneedling.
- To avoid adverse events like dyspigmentation and scarring after microneedling in skin of color, the authors recommend diligent UV light protection, the proper length of microneedles that correspond to the thickness/thinness of the targeted location on the face, and

the avoidance of excessive pressure over bony areas of the face.

- Combination treatment of microneedling with PRP shows exponential enhancement and improvement of many conditions, including the stimulation of anti-inflammatory and antifibrotic cytokines.

8.1 Introduction

In recent years, microneedling and platelet-rich plasma (PRP) either in isolation or combination have become increasingly popular treatment modalities for acne scarring, striae, scars, pigmentary disorders, hair loss, and skin rejuvenation. Particularly in skin of color, microneedling may offer a potentially safer treatment option compared to ablative and non-ablative lasers for skin resurfacing where postinflammatory hyperpigmentation and scarring are undesired potential side effects. In this chapter, we review current literature and offer treatment and safety recommendations for these modalities in skin of color.

8.2 Basic Science

8.2.1 Objective Differences in Different Ethnic Skin Types

According to the United States Census Bureau, America's diversity continues to increase with all racial and ethnic minority groups growing at faster rates than whites. With this increase in multicultural diversity in the U.S., idealistic ethnocentric variability has not only changed the standards of beauty but also the number and types of cosmetic procedures performed on skin of color patients. As such, research continues to expand our understanding of the intrinsic differences in ethnic skin, the unique

properties of its structure and function, including the amount of melanin, activity of melanocytes, variation in skin thickness, as well as fibroblastic and mast cell features, differences in pH levels, variable blood vessel reactivity, and a host of other factors currently being researched (▶ Table 8.1).[1]

Table 8.1 objective differences in skin structure in physiology based on race

Evidence supports	Insufficient evidence[a] for	Inconclusive
• Increased melanin content and melanosomal dispersion in persons of color	Racial differences in: • Skin elastic recovery/extensibility • Skin microflora • Facial for size[b]	Racial differences in: • TEWL • Water content • Corneocyte desquamation • Lipid content
• Multinucleated and larger fibroblasts in black persons compared with white persons		
• pH black < white skin		
• Larger mast cell granules, increased PLS, and increased tryptase localized to PLS in black compared with white skin		
• Variable racial blood vessel reactivity		

Abbreviations: PLS, parallel-linear striations; YEWL, transepidermal water loss.
Source: Adapted from Wesley NO, Maibach HI. Racial (ethnic) differences in skin properties: the objective data. Am J Clin Dermatol 2003;4:843–880.
[a]Scan elastic recovery/extensibility, skin microflora, and poor size or labeled as "insufficient evidence for" racial differences rather than inconclusive because only two studies are fewer examine the variables.
[b]Sugiyana-Nakagiri Y, Sugata K, Hachiya A, et al. Ethnic differences in the structural properties of facial skin. J Dermatol Sci 2009;53:135–139.

8.2.2 Melanocyte Distribution and its Relationship to Skin of Color

By far, the melanin content accounts for one of the most significant differences between persons with lighter versus darker skin types. This characteristic reflects both the quantitative and qualitative activity of the melanocytes. Within the cytoplasm of melanocytes are melanosomes that serve as the site for melanin production. Melanosomes are transferred to surrounding keratinocytes, thereby giving patients their characteristic "skin color." The size, number, and accumulation of melanosomes within each keratinocyte further contribute to the differences in complexion. Larger melanosomes with abundant melanin are singly dispersed and degraded at slower rates, contributing to darker skin seen among patients characterized as Fitzpatrick skin types (FST) III to VI. In contrast, smaller collections of melanosomes with decreased amounts of melanin contribute to lighter skin colors among patients characterized as FST I to II.[1] Additionally, melanosomes are dispersed throughout all of the layers of the epidermis in skin of color, whereas they are confined to the basal and lower malphigian layer of the epidermis in Caucasian skin.[2]

Findings from molecular genetics also support variations in ethnic skin types with defined pigmentation genes such as tyrosinase-related protein family members. Tyrosinase-related protein 1 increases tyrosinase activity and subsequently, leads to an increase in both melanin synthesis and melanosome size. Together, the aforementioned components help to explain the differences in response to ultraviolet (UV) light among different ethnicities. Likewise, melanocyte-stimulating hormone triggers the production of DNA repair proteins, which aid in

the otection of darker skinned ethnicities when exposed to damaging UV sources. Moreover, the melanocortin-1-receptor aids in the type of melanin produced by melanocytes (pheomelanin, which is red–yellow in color, and eumelanin, which is brown–black in color).[1]

8.2.3 Differences in Skin Thickness in Skin of Color

Newer studies have proposed that increased numbers of cornified cell layers and lipid content help explain increased skin thickness in darker skin types. When compared to that of whites', darker skin types have increased numbers and larger sizes of fibroblasts, suggestive of active biosynthesis and turnover of collagen.[1,2] An increased number of macrophages and smaller collagen fiber bundles further contribute to increased thickness in ethnic skin.[1] These features may be relevant when considering trends in aging and need for rejuvenation.

8.2.4 Microneedling: How It Works

Percutaneous collagen induction therapy, otherwise known as microneedling, has become a popular treatment modality for numerous dermatologic conditions. Mounting evidence shows a role for microneedling in the management of acne and other scars, hair loss, striae, pigmentary alterations, and rhytides (rejuvenation and resurfacing).[3,4] Microneedling instruments are composed of rows of fine needles that either roll over or pierce the skin to create rapidly healing microchannels, with negligible injury to the epidermis, that separate bundles of collagen while concurrently stimulating the production of new collagen and elastin.[3] The dermal microchannels stimulate a cascade of inflammatory events including the release of fibroblast growth factor, platelet-derived growth factor (PDGF), and transforming growth factor α and β (TGF-α and TGF-β).[3] Subsequent fibroblast proliferation and migration result in the formation of new blood vessels and collagen, with the creation of a fibronectin network that serves as a matrix for both type III, and eventually type I collagen deposition.[3] For more detailed information on the mechanism of action of microneedling, please refer to Chapter 5.

Lasers (both fractional and nonfractional, ablative and non-ablative), chemical peels, and dermabrasion procedures have traditionally been employed for skin resurfacing. Though effective, adverse effects including scarring, postinflammatory pigmentary changes (hyper- and hypopigmentation), and prolonged recovery time, even with fractionated non-ablative lasers, have been seen, making them higher risk procedures for patients with skin of color. Microneedling has the advantage of piercing the skin while keeping the epidermis partially intact, thus resulting in an accelerated healing process with decreased risks for scarring and infections, as opposed to fully ablative procedures. The fact that microneedling involves no thermal energy and has no specific targeted chromophores is an added benefit because there is negligible risk of incidental thermal damage to melanocytes resulting in altered pigmentation.[5]

There are a wide range of both electric-powered pen devices and fixed needle rollers that are used for microneedling with variable needle lengths, diameter, quantity, configuration, and material. Both function by smoothly rolling over the skin with a goal end point of fine pinpoint bleeding. The electrical pens have easily adjustable operating speeds and penetration depths. The electrical pens also have disposable needle tips that lower the risk of infection and allow for treatment of focal traumatic scars which is an advantage over the roller drum.[3]

To achieve desired clinical outcomes, one must consider the location of treatment and appropriate needle depth. Understanding the relative differences in skin site, contour, and thickness help to optimize device selection and depth for different cosmetic procedures. Richard and colleagues examined 15 skin biopsy specimens from different facial sites on 3 fresh adult cadavers to determine the absolute relative values of skin thickness. As depicted in ▶ Table 8.2, the upper eyelid proved to have the thinnest skin of all sites examined compared to skin at other sites measuring at least twice as thick, with the nasal tip measuring three times the thickness of the upper eyelid. Findings of relative facial skin thickness have also been reillustrated on a facial map in (▶ Fig. 8.1).[4] Therefore, deeper needle penetration, 1.5 to 3.0 mm, will be required for thicker sebaceous skin, such as the cheeks, perioral regions, and scars or striae in various body parts. Comparatively, thinner skin in the periocular regions, forehead, and nasal bridge warrant needle depths ranging from 0.5 to 1.5 mm. It is important to note that the exact needle length may not correlate with the exact depth of penetration into the skin. For example, in one study devices that exceeded 1.0 mm in depth revealed a penetration depth that was lower than anticipated.[3] Therefore, there may be a discrepancy between a needle with increased length and the exact length it penetrates into the dermis. As such, we recommend assessing for pinpoint bleeding as an endpoint compared to trying to attain a particular level of depth penetration.

Table 8.2 Relative skin thickness index

Site	Relative skin thickness index (± SD)
Upper lip	2.261 +0.539
Lower lip	2.259 +0.537
Philtrum	2.260 +0.375
Chin	3.144 +0.464
Upper eyelid	1 +0.000
Lower eyelid	2.189 +0.475
Forehead	2.850 +0.599
Right cheek	2.967 +0.661
Left cheek	3.226 +0.628
Malar eminence	2.783 +1.082
Submental	2.403 +0.500
Nasal tip	3.302 +0.491
Nasal dorsum	2.020 +0.478
Right neck	1.497 +0.824
Left neck	1.530 +0.764

Source: Adapted from Ha RY, Nojima K, Adams WP Jr., and Brown SA. Analysis of Facial Skin Thickness: Defining the Relative Thickness Index. Plast Reconstr Surg. 2005 May; 115(6):1769–73.[13]

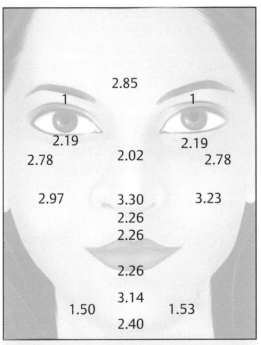

Fig. 8.1 Map of skin thickness on different parts of the face. While differences in skin thickness on the face of Caucasian skin versus skin of color is not known, it should be noted that studies have reported larger and more multinucleated fibroblasts in black versus white skin potentially resulting in differences in skin thickness. Note: ethnic/racial background of the subjects is not noted in the study that obtained these measurements. (Adapted from Ha RY, Nojima K, Adams WP Jr., and Brown SA. Analysis of Facial Skin Thickness: Defining the Relative Thickness Index. Plast Reconstr Surg. 2005 May; 115(6):1769-73.)

Almost universally, estheticians may microneedle up to 0.2 to 0.25 mm in depth, which is to but not through the stratum corneum in all ethnic skin types, thus following the guidelines of being prohibited from performing any medical treatment. Microneedling devices with needles longer than 0.3 mm are classified as a class I medical device. As such, only licensed medical professionals, such as registered nurses, nurse practitioners, physician assistants, acupuncturists, and physicians, are allowed to microneedle at depths of that length or higher. Of note, needles with a longer length tend to result in longer downtimes. Currently available microneedling devices include the Eclipse Micropen (0.5–2.0 mm) and the MD Derma Dermapen (0.25–2.5 mm).[3]

The stratum corneum continues to serve as one of the main obstacles to percutaneous absorption given it restricts the transient dermal delivery of topicals, including topical medications. Skin penetration can either be enhanced physically or chemically. Recently it has been shown that higher transdermal penetration can be seen on microneedle-injected sites. The microchannels created in the stratum corneum allow topicals to pass through and increased blood perfusion also results in increased delivery through the skin.[6] Vitamins A, C, and hyaluronic acid are vital in the assembly of new collagen.

Thus combining microneedling with topical antioxidants, hyaluronic acid, or platelet-rich plasma (PRP), may aid in the enhancement of microneedling-induced wound healing. Priming the skin with topical prior to microneedling may also help to upsurge gene and protein expression that results in skin regeneration.[3,6] It is recommended by the authors that any topical applied to the skin immediately pre- or post-microneedling be of a sterile nature as to avoid infection or biofilm formation.

8.2.5 Platelet-Rich Plasma: How It Works

Platelet rich plasma (PRP) is prepared by centrifuging a patient's blood to produce a highly concentrated autologous solution of plasma with platelet concentrations of three to five times the amount found in the patient's serum.[7,8] The platelets will then release numerous growth factors including platelet-derived growth factor (PDGF), transforming growth factor (TGF-α and TGF-β, vascular endothelial growth factor (VEGF), and many others that stimulate the healing process via cell proliferation, differentiation, and migration.[7,8,9,10, 11,12,13,14] In addition, several proteins including fibrin, fibronectin, and vitronectin are included in PRP which help to provide structural support that is necessary for cell migration. As a result, increased fibroblasts and collagen contribute to the regenerative processes that are responsible for skin rejuvenation, scar revision, treatment of alopecia, and several other dermatologic conditions.[7,10,11] For a more in-depth background on the basic science of PRP, please see Chapters 2 and 3.

8.2.6 Summary

Melanin serves as a significant filter to block the damaging effects of UV light in darker skin types. However, melanocytes and ethnic skin show labile responses o cutaneous injury making conditions such as postinflammatory pigmentary changes, acne scarring, and melasma more common.[1,2] Recently microneedling and PRP have been introduced into the armamentarium of cosmetic treatments used on ethnic skin.[1] Both are safer and effective therapeutic options as aesthetic treatments (whose properties may be augmented when combined together) with versatility and practicality for use on ethnic skin.[5,9,12]

8.3 Microneedling

8.3.1 Skin Rejuvenation

As the demands for less aggressive yet effective cosmetic procedures continue to increase, recent data has shown microneedling to be effective for facial rejuvenation treating both photodamaged skin and rhytides. While genetics, behavior, gravity, and UV exposure substantially affect the overall aging process, these changes often happen at a slower rate and "later-in-life" in darker compared to fair skinned individuals. Caucasians tend to show more signs of photoaging in their fourth decade, while darker ethnic patients may not manifest signs until their fifth or sixth decade.[1] This fact is in part potentially due to increased epidermal melanin and increased fibroblasts in the dermis in ethnic patients compared to their age-matched lighter-skinned counterparts, as described above. Darker skin types exhibit fewer rhytides than Caucasians but will often develop roughly textured skin and mottled pigmentation as a result of photoaging.[1]

However, there are fewer options for or higher risks when combating signs of photoaging. The risk of scarring and dyspigmentation results in less frequent use of ablative resurfacing for skin rejuvenation in ethnic patients. Posttreatment dyspigmentation after non-ablative resurfacing procedures is also a concern.[1] Multiple articles site microneedling as an effective treatment for rhytides and skin rejuvenation[2] Increased amounts of types I, III, and VII collagen and tropoelastin were found after six microneedling sessions in one study. Six months later, type I collagen and elastin persisted and no change in the number of melanocytes after the procedure was noted.[15,16] The increased reorganized collagen and elastic fibers in the dermis are responsible for decreased rhytides and skin tightening observed in patients.[2,15,16] A 9-year retrospective analysis looked at 480 patients who underwent one to four microneedling sessions and achieved 60 to 80% clinical improvement when compared to baseline.[17] With regards to microneedling and rejuvenation in skin of color, there may be a lag time of up to 2 months from the start of treatment to view clinically apparent results. The recommended protocol for a treatment series is three to six biweekly or monthly microneedling sessions for facial skin to fully achieve optimal results in skin rejuvenation in skin of color.[2] For the body, sessions may need to be 4 to 8 weeks apart to allow for sufficient healing time.

8.3.2 Acne Scarring

Acne scarring and pigment changes that ensue as a result of acne vulgaris can have a dramatic impact on patients' self-esteem and quality of life.[18,19] Although significant advancements have been made in the development of laser resurfacing and its use on darker-skinned

patients, microneedling has become a safer alternative compared to ablative or nonablative resurfacing, because microneedling does not emit significant amounts of thermal energy (heat), which can cause postinflammatory pigmentary changes and scarring.[1,2] It mimics fractionated non-ablative laser therapy except with mechanical injury only.

Several studies demonstrate statistically significant improvement in acne scars among all or specifically darker skin types with microneedling as monotherapy but with fewer reports of postprocedure pigmentary alteration.[18,20] Cachaferio et al conducted an evaluator-blinded randomized clinical trial in which 46 patients with atrophic acne scars underwent either non-ablative fractional erbium 1,340-nm laser versus microneedling (device: Dr. Roller, 192 microneedles, 2 mm length). While both groups demonstrated promising clinical results, 13.6% of the patients treated with laser therapy experienced postinflammatory hyperpigmentation, compared to no patients in the microneedling group.[18] In another study, 30 patients of FST IV to V with acne scars received five monthly microneedling sessions (device: Dermaroller, 192 microneedles, 1.5 mm length, 0.5 mm diameter). Photographs showed significant improvement of the scars with five patients (16.67%) developing postinflammatory hyperpigmentation, which gradually resolved in two of the patients after strict SPF compliance. The other three were lost to follow-up, so resolution was unknown. Hence, while postinflammatory pigmentary alteration can occur with microneedling, these studies and the authors' experience demonstrate clear advantages of microneedling as a cost effective, repeatable, and relatively safe treatment for skin regeneration and scar reduction.[21]

8.3.3 Pigmentary Disorders

Melasma

Microneedling has also been explored as monotherapy and as a means of transdermal drug delivery in ethnic skin for the treatment of disorders of hyperpigmentation.[2] Medium to dark brown patches on sun exposed areas, namely the forehead, cheeks, nose, upper lip, and rarely the neck or forearms, are the hallmarks of melasma. While the exact etiology is unknown, genetics; UV radiation (and to a lesser extent, infrared and visible light); as well as hormonal shifts such as those occurring during pregnancy or from contraceptive pills, hormonal replacement therapy, and even antiseizure medications may all play a role in the development of this acquired disorder.[22,23] In addition to UV radiation itself, photo-induced hormones, growth factors, and chemical mediators of inflammation, including interleukins (IL-1a, IL-1b, and IL-6), tumor necrosis factor α, eicosanoids (prostaglandins [PGs] D2, E2, F2, and leukotriene B4), and histamine, influence the function of melanocytes directly or indirectly and may further contribute to pigmentary effects of UV light.[1,24,25] Topical lightening agents, chemical peels, dermabrasion, certain laser procedures, and even off-label systemic therapies have been explored but often with partial, temporary or unsatisfactory results.[22,23] Incidental skin lightening noted during microneedling treatment for the correction of photodamage and acne scars has led to its use as monotherapy for melasma, yet there are few published studies, most with unimpressive or modest results.[26]

In contrast, when used in combination with depigmenting agents, to enhance penetration, microneedling has proven to be advantageous. Recent studies have shown that topical tranexamic acid, inhibits UV-induced plasmin activity in keratinocytes by preventing the binding of plasminogen to the keratinocytes, which ultimately results in less free arachidonic acids and a diminished ability to produce PGs and thus, decreases melanocyte tyrosinase activity.[25] A randomized study of 60 patients with moderate to severe melasma (FST IV–V), compared microneedling plus topical tranexamic acid 4 mg/mL application (microneedling device: 192 microneedles, 1.5 mm length, 0.25 mm diameter) versus TA 4 mg/mL microinjections (100 U/mL insulin syringe with a 4 mm mesoneedle at 1 cm interval injections). There was 44% improvement in the microneedling group versus 35% in the microinjections group, a statistically significant difference after just 3 sessions per the Melasma area severity index (MASI) score. Furthermore, at least 50% improvement was seen in 41.38% of patients in the microneedling compared to 26.09% in the microinjection group. There were no adverse effects noted through the duration of this study.[2,5,22] In another trial investigating transcutaneous drug delivery via microneedling, Fabbrocini et al conducted a split-faced study of 20 women with melasma (FST III–V) who underwent microneedling (microneedling device: Derma-roller-Model CIT 8, which consists of 192 needles, needle length of 0.5 mm, and a diameter of 0.02 mm arranged in an array on a roller device) followed by application of a depigmenting serum with rucinol (a tyrosinase inhibitor) and sophora α (an α-MSH inhibitor) versus the depigmenting serum alone. After 2 months, the microneedling group improved by 10.1 points on the MASI score, while the non-microneedling group only improved by 7.1 points.[5,6] MASI score < 10 was mild; 10 to 15 was moderate; and > 15 was severe (▶ Fig. 8.2).[27] The luminance index scores, a colorimetric evaluation that can objectively measure the expression of brightness in skin pigment, were also statistically significant ($p < 0.05$) in the patients that received combination therapy, with an increased brightness of 17.4%.[2,6]

Periorbital Melanosis

Periorbital melanosis is an often idiopathic, cosmetically displeasing condition characterized as homogeneous darkly pigmented round patches encompassing the periorbital rim (usually infraorbitally), as depicted in ▶ Fig. 8.3.[28,29] Cur-

rent treatments include avoidance and treatment of potential allergens, application of topical retinoids and/or lightening agents, chemical peels, filler injection into the tear trough area, and certain laser therapies. Nevertheless, results are often suboptimal.[28]

Combination microneedling procedures may be an effective and innovative treatment option for this condition.[2,28] Sahni and Kassir reported a 48-year-old man (FST V) with severe, idiopathic periorbital melanosis who underwent treatment with the DermaFrac device (0.25-mm tip-cap at a pressure of 10 mm Hg), which uses microneedling, along with a vacuum-assisted infusion of a serum containing antiaging (containing

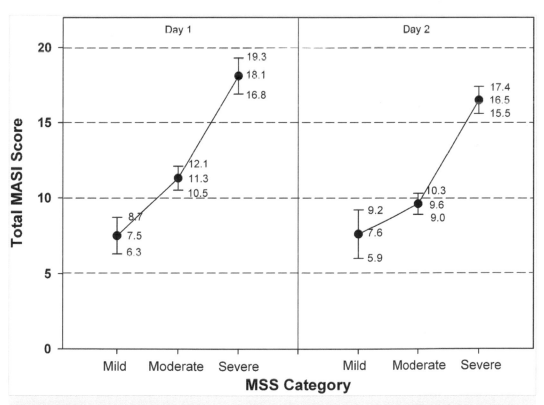

Fig. 8.2 Melasma area severity index provides representation for entry scores for patients with moderate to severe melasma. (Adapted from Pandya et al.[27] Reliability assessment and validation of the Melasma Area and Severity Index (MASI) and a new modified MASI scoring method. JAAD. 2011; 64(1); 78–83.)

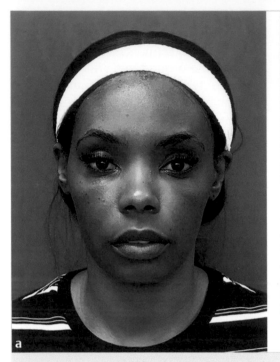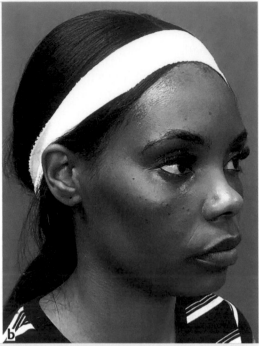

Fig. 8.3 (a, b) A 30-year-old female patient (Fitzpatrick skin type V) complained of periorbital melanosis and noticeable tear troughs. She subsequently underwent two different procedures: (1) PRP injection to tear troughs, and (2) microneedling with PRP for periorbital melanosis and skin rejuvenation.

meristoyl pentapeptide 17 sympeptide, acetyl octapeptide-3 SNAP 8, palmitoyl pentapeptide-4 matrixyl, acetyl hexapeptide-8 argirilene and tripeptide syn-ake), and lightening (kojic acid) compounds.[28] Physician global assessment scoring (PGA) revealed 50 to 75% and 75 to 90% improvement after 4 and 12 sessions, respectively, with no reported side effects. The investigators hypothesized benefits resulted from improved skin hydration and induction of collagen and elastin synthesis, processes that diminish the visibility of dermal pigment.[2,28] In another study, 13 women with mild to severe periorbital melanosis were treated with microneedling followed by topical application of 10% trichloroacetic acid (TCA) for 5 minutes. Almost all patients showed significant aesthetic improvement with a fair, good, or excellent response in 92.3% using both a patient and physician global assessment tool. Only mild discomfort, transient erythema, and edema were noted both during and immediately after the procedure. There was also no recurrence of the dark circles up to 4 months after the procedure.[29]

It is important to note that dermal melanocytosis, allergic dermatitis, pigmentary demarcation lines, excessive subcutaneous vascularity, hormonal abnormalities, shadowing due to skin laxity, and tear troughs associated with aging may all contribute to periorbital melanosis. Therefore, it is critical to understand the different contributing factors and address each appropriately; often a combination approach is most optimal and microneedling may enhance penetration of depigmenting agents, making it an easy, effective booster to in-office therapies.[28]

8.3.4 Striae

Striae distensae, colloquially referred to as stretch marks, are atrophic linear plaques in the dermal layer, most often found on the breasts, abdomen, hips, and thighs, due to disruption of the collagen-elastic matrix during the adolescent growth spurt or pregnancy or from hormonal and weight changes.[30] Though rarely medically concerning, striae can cause significant emotional distress. Microneedling may help ameliorate stretch marks by stimulating keratinocytes to release growth factors that promote collagen deposition and extracellular matrix remodeling. A study of 16 patients, FST III to IV, with striae distensae, showed improvement on both physician and patient assessment grading scales. The physician grading scale was a quartile grading system (0: change, 0%; 1: minimal improvement, <25%; 2: moderate improvement, 26–50%; 3: marked improvement, 51–75%; 4: excellent improvement, 76–100%). Excellent improvement was seen among seven patients (43.8%) after three monthly treatments of microneedling (DTS roller; DTS-MG, Inc., Seoul, Korea; 1.5 mm needle depth). The additional nine patients showed minimal to moderate improvement. Patient satisfaction scores revealed 37.5% patients were highly satisfied, 50.0% somewhat satisfied, and 12.5% unsatisfied. Minor side effects included mild pain, erythema, and spotty bleeding during and after the treatments.[5,31] Another study compared microneedling to microdermabrasion with sonopheresis among 40 women, FST III to IV, with striae distensae. There was statistically significant clinical improvement after microneedling compared to microdermabrasion. Increased epidermal thickening, fibroblast, and collagen were seen in 90% of microneedling-treated patients versus 50% of microdermabrasion patients.[32] In another trial, while both groups demonstrated increased fibroblasts and epidermal thickness at 6 months in a randomized, evaluator-blinded trial of 20 Egyptian women with striae distensae treated with either microneedling versus fractional CO_2 laser, 90% of microneedling patients achieved significant improvement versus only 50% in the laser group.[31] Another important factor to consider when treating striae distensae is the fact that microneedling may be safe on the body in regions where laser treatment or deep peelings cannot be performed given increased risk of side effects.[30]

8.3.5 Adverse Events and Safety Considerations

It is advisable to evaluate patients' skin type, desired areas of treatment, and skin quality and texture prior to any cosmetic procedure. Several contraindications of particular importance in all patients include inflammatory acne or infections within the treatment area to minimize the introduction of microabscesses or granulomas into the skin, particularly in patients who are immunosuppressed. A predisposition for keloid development should also be discussed as it may be a contraindication to microneedling. History of oral herpes labialis should lend to pretreatment prophylaxis with oral antiviral medications such as valacyclovir prior to treatment.

Microneedling therapy can be safely performed on all skin colors and types with less risk of dyspigmentation, which is a major safety feature distinguishing it from other invasive procedures used to treat wrinkles and depressed scars, such as laser resurfacing, deep chemical peels, and dermabrasion.[33] Minor procedural pain, postprocedure erythema, pinpoint bleeding, and bruising are common adverse events, as reported in some of the small studies discussed in this chapter. In regards to skin of color (FST IV–VI), dyspigmentation after microneedling was once considered high risk. However, this complication can often be avoided with diligent UV light protection. A histologic analysis of skin melanocytes 24 hours after microneedling demonstrated neither change in melanocyte number nor any epidermal disruption.[18] It has also been shown that the up-regulation of IL-10 after microneedling exerts a suppressor activity and down-regulates melanocyte-stimulating hormone. Hence, there is a lower risk of dyspigmentation status post-microneedling, which can be safely performed among darker skin types.[19]

Scarring is still a concern with microneedling in skin of color, especially if there is excessive trauma. Pahwa et al described a 25-year-old woman who developed multiple discrete papular scars in both the horizontal and vertical direction similar to a "tram-tracks" over the temporal area, zygomatic arch, and forehead after two needling treatments (spaced 5 months apart). The microneedling device used weighed 18 g with 192 needles; 2 mm in length spaced 2 mm apart. She also reported pain during the procedure, edema, transient erythema, and postinflammatory hyperpigmentation. The authors postulated that the large size of the device or stronger pressures used during treatment may have caused her scarring. Two patients from a microneedling study of 32 men and women, FST IV to V (device: Dermaroller, 192 needles 1.5 mm in length) also developed tram-track scar that improved by 20 to 30% in one subject after 3 months of topical tretinoin 0.025% gel.[21] To minimize these and other risks, we recommended avoiding excessive pressure over bony areas of the face, such as the forehead and nose, particularly among patients with skin of color, since increased bruising in these areas more often leads to hyperpigmentation. Also, use microneedles that are smaller than or equal to 2.0 mm in length.[34] In areas with thin skin such as the upper face, periorbital region, and neck, shorter length needles (i.e., 1.0 mm) may be even safer.

8.4 Fractional Radiofrequency Microneedling

Another technique for facial rejuvenation and the treatment of acne scars involves using radiofrequency (RF)-emitting microneedles. The motivation behind development and appeal of such devices is their ability to deliver energy at precise depths in an effort to stimulate collagen remodeling, skin tightening, and even reduction of fat depending on the depth of penetration.[35] Fractional radiofrequency microneedling (FRFM) results in mechanical disruption of dermal fibrotic strands that lead to the downward skin retraction giving atrophic scars their appearance. RF energy delivered dermally promotes collagen remodeling to replace scar tissue with new healthier pliable fibers.[36] There are monopolar or bipolar RF, and insulated or non-insulated microneedle RF microneedling systems. An in depth discussion of RF microneedling systems is described in Chapter 7. With regards to skin of color, RF microneedling systems using insulation along most of the needle shaft, leaving only a small part of the tips non-insulated, may be preferable. This insulation protects the collateral epidermis from heating and thus damage, but sometimes requires multiple passes with different depths to cover several layers of the tissue. Additionally, they may produce micro-bruises with many bleeding points on the surface of the skin, because there is no coagulation at the upper skin layers.

Other, non-insulated RF microneedling systems allow for coagulation along the entire length of the needle and minimize microbleeds during treatment. Non-insulated needles result in the RF flowing through all dermal layers at one time allowing 7 to 10 times larger tissue volume to be treated.[34] but risk of thermal injury to the epidermis is also higher. Therefore, non-insulated RF microneedles may lead to increased incidence of scarring and postinflammatory pigmentary alteration and should be used with caution particularly in skin of color, unless other device designs to protect epidermis (burying the needle, temperature control, etc.) have been implemented.

FRFM devices may have an advantage over traditional fractional laser devices because they deliver energy more selectively, given the fixed spacing and depth of each needle, and may be able to address fat and cellulite depending on the depth of penetration.[3] Examples of FRFM systems include the INFINI,[33] Profound, Vivace, Endymed Intensif RF, and Secret RF microneedling devices (most of which are insulated systems).

8.4.1 Skin Rejuvenation

FRFM has been studied for skin rejuvenation in ethnic patients.[3] Fifteen women with FST III to IV underwent a split-face trial in which half of their faces received FRFM (non-insulated fractional RF device, Scarlet, Viol Co., Korea) alone and the other half combination of FRFM and stem cell conditioned medium. After three treatment sessions, both sides of the face showed improvements in hydration, erythema index, and skin roughness. The addition of the stem cell medium

produced a statistically significant improvement in fine wrinkles and overall appearance compared with FRFM alone (2.20 ± 0.68 vs. 2.06 ± 0.70; $p < 0.05$). Side effects were limited to procedural pain and transient erythema.[37]

8.4.2 Acne Scars

There are several trials showing benefits of FRFM on acne scars in darker skin types.[38] A study of 19 patients comparing the efficacy and safety of FRFM for acne scars in patients with FST III to V after 3 monthly sessions showed not only a 47% improvement in dyschromia but also an improvement of at least 1 acne scar grade, according to the Goodman and Baron's global qualitative acne scarring system. One patient did develop postinflammatory hyperpigmentation that spontaneously resolved after 4 weeks.[36] Cho et al demonstrated not only 73% improvement in acne scars after just two sessions among 30 patients but also reduction in enlarged pores among 70% of participants. Of note, the authors did not comment on FTS but practice in Seoul, Korea so presumably included at least some patients of Asian descent. While some reported temporary roughness, the skin softened after 8 weeks of treatment.[38] Another study of 31 patients, FTS III to V, with moderate to severe acne scars underwent four FRFM treatments 6 weeks apart. All 31 demonstrated improvement (3% had very good improvement, 9% had good improvement, 58% had moderate improvement, and 29% had minimal improvement) with only transient erythema and postinflammatory hyperpigmentation after the procedure.[39] While FRFM does require multiple treatments with modified settings based on FST, evidence confirms improvement in acne scars among darker skin type patients with minimal downtime and chronic dyspigmentation sequela.[36,38,39]

8.5 Platelet-Rich Plasma

8.5.1 PRP Quality, Concentrations, and Differences in Ethnic Skin

During the preparation of this chapter, we performed a literature search for ethnic differences in PRP. There are no trials published to date on this specific subject. However, one study including 75 black or white subjects (16 of whom had sickle cell trait) showed that reduced platelet aggregation and/or low concentrations of ristocetin is a normal finding in many blacks. They also found that these differences are not related to the presence of sickle hemoglobin as originally hypothesized and appears to result from the presence of a plasma inhibitor against RIPA. Whether or not a plasma inhibitor against RIPA would affect concentrations or quality of PRP for cosmetic rejuvenation or hair growth is unknown, but an interesting difference to consider when understanding possible ethnic differences in PRP in future studies.[40]

8.5.2 Concentration of PRP and Effects on Potential Efficacy

There have been no reports of differences in efficacy of PRP in ethnic patients versus Caucasian patients. However, different biological responses are seen as a result of the wide variation in reported protocols on how to obtain PRP in general.[8] Time, centrifugal acceleration, and the distance between the particles are all key factors that contribute to the quality and efficacy. In addition, the rotor to the volume of processed white blood cells, prevention of platelet aggregation, and minimization of the platelet gradient are all relative aspects that can affect the efficacy of PRP.[8] Efficient conditions for platelet recovery are low centrifugal acceleration (close to 100 × g, 10 minutes) in the first spin and around 400 × g in the second spin for preventing effects on activating platelets.[8]

8.5.3 PRP with Microneedling

Clinicians have most recently incorporated the use of PRP with the aim of augmenting cosmetic aesthetic outcomes.[9] Combining increased collagen deposition, elastic fiber formation, and dermal thickness seen as a result of microneedling, with the regenerative effects of growth factors within highly concentrated PRP, aim to make the skin function as if it were younger and maintain its youthful properties. Combination treatment is described as PRP applied to the treatment areas followed by microneedling over it to drive the PRP into desired locations.[10] By combining both procedures, studies have shown the exponential enhancement and improvement of acne scars, skin rejuvenation, and even hair loss.[12] This is in part due to microneedling creating perforations that increase PRP absorption and the capability of the platelets to contribute to wound healing prompted by microneedling. Recently microarray studies have found that microneedling up regulates the expression of TGF-β3, which is an essential marker in the prevention of scarring given its antifibrotic properties.[12]

Several studies including darker FST have provided evidence of the advantages microneedling has with PRP compared to just microneedling alone. Asif et al completed a split-face comparison study of 50 patients (FST III–V) with atrophic acne scars comparing microneedling plus intradermal injections and the topical application of PRP versus microneedling plus intradermal injections of distilled water. Scars treated by both modalities improved by 62% versus single therapy only improving by 45%. Together microneedling plus PRP resulted in 40% excellent improvement and 60% good improvement in patients in this study.[10,11] Fabbrocini et al also did a split-face study in which they evaluated 12 patients and compared microneedling plus PRP to microneedling alone for the treatment of acne scars. While the acne scars improved on both sides of the face, there was a significantly greater reduction and scar severity on the side treated with microneedling plus PRP.[12] The exact FST was not noted in this study, but the study was done at the University of Naples Federico II (in Napoli NA, Italy), so it is presumed that some of the patients with FST

III+ were included in the study. Ibrahim and colleagues also demonstrated the effects of combining PRP with microneedling for the treatment of atrophic scars based on comparisons of three study groups (FST II–IV) treated with either microneedling alone (28 patients), PRP alone (34 patients), or microneedling plus PRP (28 patients). Of note, the device used for microneedling was the Dermapen 3, with 9 microneedles of 0.25 to 2.5 mm length. All three groups showed a reduction in the score associated with the clinical evaluation scale for atrophic scarring, as well as statistically significant improvement in the appearance of the atrophic acne scars. This was further supported by the development of increased rete ridges in the epidermis posttreatment (▶ Fig. 8.4a, b). Elastic fibers also increased posttreatment as a result of

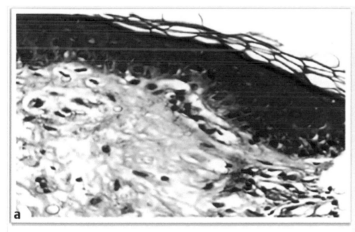

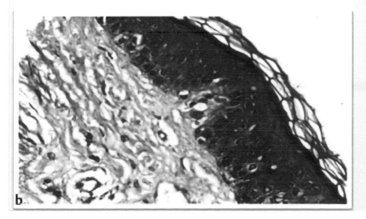

Fig. 8.4 (a) Histologic image showing an acne scar with a thin epidermis and flattened rete ridges prior to treatment with microneedling and platelet-rich plasma (H&E 9400). (b) Histologic imaging showing an acne scar after treatment with a thickened epidermis and normal rete ridges (H&E 9400).

both PRP and microneedling treatment (▶ Fig. 8.5a, b). The improvement was most obvious in group three supporting evidence for combined treatment with microneedling and PRP. There were no reports of hyper- or hypopigmentation seen in any of the patients, both Caucasian and darker skinned patients.[14]

Recently El-Doymati and colleagues reported that microneedling combined with PRP were superior to microneedling monotherapy for the treatment of atrophic acne scars in a split face study.[41] There were 24 subjects in the study, 21 which had FST IV and the remaining FST III. The subjects were split into three groups: group A subjects were treated with combined microneedling and PRP on one side of the face and microneedling alone on the opposite side; group B subjects were treated with combined microneedling and TCA 15% on one side and microneedling alone on the other side of the face; group C subjects were treated with combined microneedling and PRP versus combined microneedling and TCA 15% on opposite sides of the face. The microneedling device was Dermaroller (ADROLL, TD, Spain) with 600 stainless steel needles and a needle length of 1.5 mm. Both photography and punch biopsies were utilized for clinical and pathologic evaluation. At the conclusion of the study, combined therapy with either microneedling and PRP or microneedling and TCA showed significant

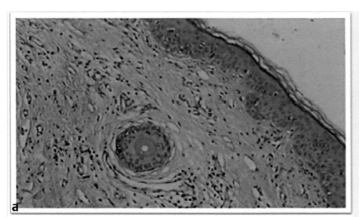

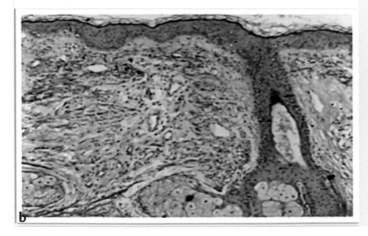

Fig. 8.5 (a) Histologic image showing an acne scar before microneedling and PRP with scanty fragmented elastic fibers (Orcein 9100). (b) Histologic image showing an acne scar post-treatment with increased elastic fibers (Orcein 9100).

improvement when compared with microneedling as monotherapy or atrophic acne scars ($p=0.015$ and 0.011, respectively).[41] An interesting observation with this study is that microneedling combined with TCA was superior to microneedling and PRP combination therapy in skin of color. The addition of TCA not only improved the skin texture but also aided in the induction of collagenesis and may serve as a superior option for acne scar treatment in skin of color. ► Fig. 8.3 and ► Fig. 8.6, ► Fig. 8.7, and ► Fig. 8.8 depict the clinical picture of combining microneedling with PRP for the treatment of periorbital melanosis and skin rejuvenation. **Video 8.1** also demonstrates the combined procedure of PRP with microneedling.

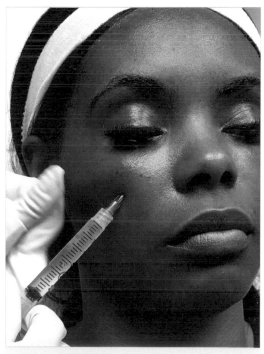

Fig. 8.6 Demonstration of platelet-rich plasma injection for periorbital melanosis, injected with 3 cc syringe and 1.5 inch 28 g cannula.

8.5.4 PRP and Hair Loss

The new trends in hair loss have shifted from traditional therapies to those that influence the stem cells at the root of the hair follicle. By focusing on the stem cells antiapoptotic effects, increased survival of the hair follicle and lengthening of the anagen phase of the hair cycle are achieved to stimulate hair growth. PRP influences the stem cells to proliferate and differentiate that will lead to an upper regulation of β-catenin and activity that stimulate hair growth by inducing the differentiation of stem cells and hair follicle cells.[10] Several studies have investigated treating various scalp conditions with PRP, especially given the indefinite nature of traditional treatments such as finasteride and minoxidil.[13] As such, nonsurgical options are becoming increasingly desirable for individuals affected by hair loss.

Nonscarring Alopecia

Multiple studies demonstrate effects of PRP on nonscarring hair loss including androgenetic alopecia and alopecia areata.[10,13,42,43,44] Based on literature review at the time of this text's publication, there are no known trials investigating specific racial/ethnic difference in response to PRP for nonscarring alopecia and many published studies fail to differentiate explicitly. After speaking with several experts in the field, it is our opinion that benefits do not differ according to overarching ethnic groups and related more to individual variables such as duration and extent of hair loss. **Video 8.2** demonstrates the procedure of scalp injections with PRP for androgenetic alopecia in Middle Eastern man with FST III skin.

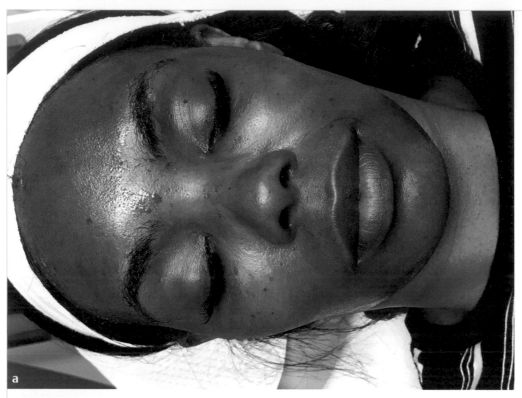

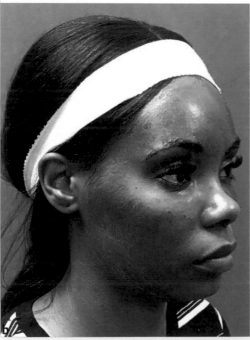

Fig. 8.7 (a,b) Images **(a)** immediately after and **(b)** 10 minutes after PRP has been left to dry, status post microneedling plus platelet-rich plasma for rejuvenation in Fitzpatrick skin type V skin.

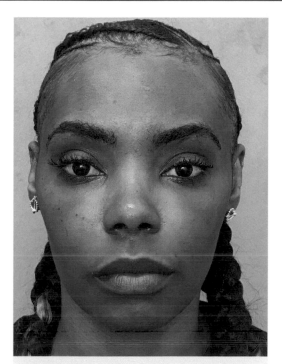

Fig. 8.8 Four days post microneedling plus platelet-rich plasma (PRP) in Fitzpatrick skin type V skin. Note mild desquamation on the forehead. Mild peeling/desquamation may last up to 1 week. Swelling from PRP tear trough injection has resolved, but improvement in tear trough and periorbital melanosis is still noted.

Scarring (Cicatricial) Alopecia

Though no rigorous clinical trials examining PRP for scarring hair loss exist, there are several case reports supporting its effects. Central centrifugal cicatricial alopecia and traction alopecia are two distressing and often disfiguring conditions that are more prevalent among patients with darker skin types. In the authors' experience, early to moderate traction hair loss prior to full obliteration of follicular ostia responds well to PRP injections, and patients using heavy hair extensions and braids have been some of our most satisfied. While PRP shows promising advances for the management of hair loss including stimulating hair growth and

increasing shaft diameter, larger clinical trials are needed to fully assess its efficacy.[10,13,45,46]

8.5.5 PRP and Skin Rejuvenation

Irrespective of FST, PRP impacts the production and remodeling of collagen type I, elastin, and hyaluronic acid as well as alters the degradation function of matrix metalloproteinases, factors that cumulatively enhance skin support, volume, elasticity, and hydration to improve skin texture, color, and tone.[10,14] Several studies have looked at PRP effects for rejuvenation in skin of color patients. Much of this literature comes from the North Africa, the Middle East, and/or Asia among subjects with FST III and IV. Kang et al published preliminary finding from a prospective, randomized split-face trial on lower eyelid skin in which 10 Asian women with wrinkling and darkened skin tone received unactivated PRP injection to the infraorbital region on one side of the face and platelet-poor plasma (PPP) to the other, while another group of 10 received PRP versus saline control. They underwent three monthly treatments with final evaluation, including photographic assessment by three blinded dermatologists, patient self-assessment and satisfaction questionnaires, and spectrophotometry for erythema and melanin indices, 3 months after the final session. PRP produced statistically significant improvement in wrinkles and skin tone compared to PPP or saline with erythema and melanin indices dropping from 8.52 to 7.37 ($p = 0.01$) and 34.42 to 31.86 ($p < 0.01$), respectively. Interestingly, two patients saw improvement with both PRP and PPP suggesting serum factors may have a role in periocular rejuvenation and pigment alteration. Immediate redness, purpura, and edema were the most common adverse effects that resolved within days of therapy. The investigators do note that four of the 20 participants were lost to follow-up for unclear reasons, so small sample size and biases may influence these favorable results seen among an Asian population.[47]

But, other uncontrolled trials support improvement in greater FST as well. Mehryan et al reported statistically significant clinical improvements in infraorbital color homogeneity and crow's feet fine lines after a single PRP treatment among 10 participants, FST III and IV. Yet, wrinkle volume and visibility, melanin content, and epidermal stratum corneum hydration did not significantly change.[48] Transient side effects included a mild burning sensation and transient bruising, which both resolved.

Another study among 20 participants, FST III and IV, receiving a single intradermal PRP injection session at the nasolabial folds, periocular region, and forehead showed statistically significant reduction in the validated Wrinkle Severity Rating Scale over 8 weeks (all sites: before, 2.90 ± 0.91 and after, 2.10 ± 0.79). The most significant results occurred among younger participants with mild to moderate wrinkles, all of whom showed a greater than 25% improvement. Furthermore, 14 of 17 subjects who had nasolabial fold treatment showed more than a 25% reduction. Skin homogeneity and texture also improved markedly ($p < 0.001$) with 35% reporting a score of 5 "improved greatly" on the Skin Homogeneity and Texture scale.[49] Consider that these studies evaluated patients at early times points after only a single therapy, whereas the most robust clinical trials confirm longer terns effects occurring at three to six months status post treatment, particular with series of injection session.

▶ Fig. 8.6 demonstrates PRP injected into the tear trough area to improve periorbital melanosis in a female patient with FST V skin. Improvement in skin color and quality can be noted both post-procedure and at day 4 as depicted in ▶ Fig. 8.7 and ▶ Fig. 8.8, despite resorption of the majority of the PRP fluid by that point.

8.5.6 Adverse Events and Safety Considerations

Though direct studies investigating racial/ethnic difference in response to PRP are lacking, there is mounting evidence suggesting PRP therapy can be safely performed on all skin colors and types with no reported cases of permanent and lower risk of transient dyspigmentation.[10,11,12,13,14] Mild procedural pain, erythema, or bruising may occur and are more likely when combined with microneedling.[12,14] A thorough exam and review of risk factors for adverse events should be conducted prior to any cosmetic procedure, which has been discussed in Chapter 10.

8.5.7 PRP Conclusion

While data confirms that PRP can be beneficial for many dermatologic applications, studies in ethnic skin are lacking. Ways to optimize formulations and applications continue to evolve, and it is necessary to gain better understanding of these principles, molecular mechanisms, and safety among patients with darker skin types. In the future, larger studies demonstrating its efficacy as well as ideal protocol recommendations will increase the implementation of PRP not only as monotherapy but as an adjunct to already well-established treatments.[13]

References

[1] Talakoub L, Wesley NO. Differences in perceptions of beauty and cosmetic procedures performed in ethnic patients. Semin Cutan Med Surg. 2009; 28(2):115–129

[2] Grimes PE, Few JW. Procedures in Cosmetic Dermatology: Soft Tissue Augmentation. Philadelphia, PA: Elsevier; 2008

[3] Alster TS, Graham PM. Microneedling: a review and practical guide. Dermatol Surg. 2018; 44(3):397–404

[4] Ha RY, Nojima K, Adams WP, Jr, Brown SA. Analysis of facial skin thickness: defining the relative thickness index. Plast Reconstr Surg. 2005; 115(6):1769–1773

[5] Cohen BE, Elbuluk N. Microneedling in skin of color: a review of uses and efficacy. J Am Acad Dermatol. 2016; 74(2):348–355

[6] Fabbrocini G, De Vita V, Fardella N, et al. Skin needling to enhance depigmenting serum penetration in the treatment of melasma. Plast Surg Int. 2011; 2011:158241

[7] Leo MS, Kumar AS, Kirit R, Konathan R, Sivamani RK. Systematic review of the use of platelet-rich plasma in aesthetic dermatology. J Cosmet Dermatol. 2015; 14(4):315–323

[8] Perez AGM, Lana JFSD, Rodrigues AA, Luzo ACM, Belangero WD, Santana MHA. Relevant aspects of centrifugation step in the preparation of platelet-rich plasma. ISRN Hematol. 2014; 2014:176060

[9] Hashim PW, Levy Z, Cohen JL, Goldenberg G. Microneedling therapy with and without platelet-rich plasma. Cutis. 2017; 99(4):239–242

[10] Elghblawi E. Plasma-rich plasma, the ultimate secret for youthful skin elixir and hair growth triggering. J Cosmet Dermatol. 2018; 17(3):423–430

[11] Asif M, Kanodia S, Singh K. Combined autologous platelet-rich plasma with microneedling verses microneedling with distilled water in the treatment of atrophic acne scars: a concurrent split-face study. J Cosmet Dermatol. 2016; 15(4):434–443

[12] Fabbrocini G, De Vita V, Pastore F, et al. Combined use of skin needling and platelet-rich plasma in acne scarring treatment. Cosmet Dermatol. 2011; 24(4):177–183

[13] Singh MK. Commentary on 'Platelet-rich plasma for androgenetic alopecia: a pilot study'. Dermatol Surg. 2014; 40(9):1020–1021

[14] Ibrahim ZA, El-Ashmawy AA, Shora OA. Therapeutic effect of microneedling and autologous platelet-rich plasma in the treatment of atrophic scars: A randomized study. J Cosmet Dermatol. 2017; 16(3):388–399

[15] Bonati LM, Epstein GK, Strugar TL. Microneedling in all skin types: a review. J Drugs Dermatol. 2017; 16(4):308–313

[16] El-Domyati M, Barakat M, Awad S, Medhat W, El-Fakahany H, Farag H. Multiple microneedling sessions for minimally invasive facial rejuvenation: an objective assessment. Int J Dermatol. 2015; 54(12):1361–1369

[17] Aust MC, Fernandes D, Kolokythas P, Kaplan HM, Vogt PM. Percutaneous collagen induction therapy: an alternative treatment for scars, wrinkles, and skin laxity. Plast Reconstr Surg. 2008; 121(4):1421–1429

[18] Cachafeiro T, Escobar G, Maldonado G, Cestari T, Corleta O. Comparison of nonablative fractional erbium laser 1,340 nm and microneedling for the treatment of atrophic acne scars: a randomized clinical trial. Dermatol Surg. 2016; 42(2):232–241

[19] Alexis AF, Coley MK, Nijhawan RI, et al. Nonablative fractional laser resurfacing for acne scarring in patients with fitzpatrick skin phototypes IV-VI. Dermatol Surg. 2016; 42(3):392–402

[20] Alam M, Han S, Pongprutthipan M, et al. Efficacy of a needling device for the treatment of acne scars: a randomized clinical trial. JAMA Dermatol. 2014; 150(8):844–849

[21] Dogra S, Yadav S, Sarangal R. Microneedling for acne scars in Asian skin type: an effective low cost treatment modality. J Cosmet Dermatol. 2014; 13(3):180–187

[22] Budamakuntla L, Loganathan E, Suresh DH, et al. A randomised, open-label, comparative study of tranexamic acid microinjections and tranexamic acid with microneedling in patients with melasma. J Cutan Aesthet Surg. 2013; 6(3):139–143

[23] Lee JH, Park JG, Lim SH, et al. Localized intradermal microinjection of tranexamic acid for treatment of melasma in Asian patients: a preliminary clinical trial. Dermatol Surg. 2006; 32(5):626–631

[24] Morelli JG, Norris DA. Influence of inflammatory mediators and cytokines on human melanocyte function. J Invest Dermatol. 1993; 100(2) Suppl:191S–195S

[25] Maeda K, Naganuma M. Topical trans-4-aminomethylcyclohexanecarboxylic acid prevents ultraviolet radiation-induced pigmentation. J Photochem Photobiol B. 1998; 47(2–3):136–141

[26] Lima EdeA. Microneedling in facial recalcitrant melasma: report of a series of 22 cases. An Bras Dermatol. 2015; 90(6):919–921

[27] Pandya AG, Hynan LS, Bhore R, et al. Reliability assessment and validation of the Melasma Area and Severity Index (MASI) and a new modified MASI scoring method. J Am Acad Dermatol. 2011; 64(1):78–83, 83.e1–83.e2

[28] Sahni K, Kassir M. Dermafrac™: an innovative new treatment for periorbital melanosis in a dark-skinned male patient. J Cutan Aesthet Surg. 2013; 6(3):158–160

[29] Kontochristopoulos G, Kouris A, Platsidaki E, Markantoni V, Gerodimou M, Antoniou C. Combination of microneedling and 10% trichloroacetic acid peels in the management of infraorbital dark circles. J Cosmet Laser Ther. 2016; 18(5):289–292

[30] Aust MC, Knobloch K, Vogt PM. Percutaneous collagen induction therapy as a novel therapeutic option for Striae distensae. Plast Reconstr Surg. 2010; 126(4):219e–220e

[31] Park KY, Kim HK, Kim SE, Kim BJ, Kim MN. Treatment of striae distensae using needling therapy: a pilot study. Dermatol Surg. 2012; 38(11):1823–1828

[32] Nassar A, Ghomey S, El Gohary Y, El-Desoky F. Treatment of striae distensae with needling therapy versus microdermabrasion with sonophoresis. J Cosmet Laser Ther. 2016; 18(6):330–334

[33] Khater MH, Khattab FM, Abdelhaleem MR. Treatment of striae distensae with needling therapy versus CO2 fractional laser. J Cosmet Laser Ther. 2016; 18(2):75–79

[34] Pahwa M, Pahwa P, Zaheer A. "Tram track effect" after treatment of acne scars using a microneedling device. Dermatol Surg. 2012; 38(7 Pt 1):1107–1108

[35] Sadick N, Rothaus KO. Minimally invasive radiofrequency devices. Clin Plast Surg. 2016; 43(3):567–575

[36] Pudukadan D. Treatment of acne scars on darker skin types using a noninsulated smooth motion, electronically controlled radiofrequency microneedles treatment system. Dermatol Surg. 2017; 43 Suppl 1:S64–S69

[37] Seo KY, Kim DH, Lee SE, Yoon MS, Lee HJ. Skin rejuvenation by microneedle fractional radiofrequency and a human stem cell conditioned medium in Asian skin: a randomized controlled investigator blinded split-face study. J Cosmet Laser Ther. 2013; 15(1):25–33

[38] Cho SI, Chung BY, Choi MG, et al. Evaluation of the clinical efficacy of fractional radiofrequency microneedle treatment in acne scars and large facial pores. Dermatol Surg. 2012; 38(7 Pt 1):1017–1024

[39] Chandrashekar BS, Sriram R, Mysore R, Bhaskar S, Shetty A. Evaluation of microneedling fractional radiofrequency device for treatment of acne scars. J Cutan Aesthet Surg. 2014; 7(2):93–97

[40] Buchanan GR, Holtkamp CA, Levy EN. Racial differences in ristocetin-induced platelet aggregation. Br J Haematol. 1981; 49(3):455–464

[41] El-Domyati M, Abdel-Wahab H, Hossam A. Microneedling combined with platelet-rich plasma or trichloroacetic acid peeling for management of acne scarring: a split-face clinical and histologic comparison. J Cosmet Dermatol. 2018; 17(1):73–83

[42] Schiavone G, Raskovic D, Greco J, Abeni D. Platelet-rich plasma for androgenetic alopecia: a pilot study. Dermatol Surg. 2014; 40(9):1010–1019

[43] Giordano S, Romeo M, Lankinen P. Platelet-rich plasma for androgenetic alopecia: Does it work? Evidence from meta-analysis. J Cosmet Dermatol. 2017; 16(3):374–381

[44] Kumaran MS, Arshdeep. Platelet-rich plasma in dermatology: boon or a bane? Indian J Dermatol Venereol Leprol. 2014; 80 (1):5–14

[45] Bolanča Ž, Goren A, Getaldić-Švarc B, Vučić M, Šitum M. Platelet-rich plasma as a novel treatment for lichen planopillaris. Dermatol Ther (Heidelb). 2016; 29(4):233–235

[46] Saxena K, Saxena DK, Savant SS. Successful hair transplant outcome in cicatricial lichen planus of the scalp by combining scalp and beard hair along with platelet rich plasma. J Cutan Aesthet Surg. 2016; 9(1):51–55

[47] Kang BK, Shin MK, Lee JH, Kim NI. Effects of platelet-rich plasma on wrinkles and skin tone in Asian lower eyelid skin: preliminary results from a prospective, randomised, split-face trial. Eur J Dermatol. 2014; 24(1):100–101

[48] Mehryan P, Zartab H, Rajabi A, Pazhoohi N, Firooz A. Assessment of efficacy of platelet-rich plasma (PRP) on infraorbital dark circles and crow's feet wrinkles. J Cosmet Dermatol. 2014; 13(1):72–78

[49] Elnehrawy NY, Ibrahim ZA, Eltoukhy AM, Nagy HM. Assessment of the efficacy and safety of single platelet-rich plasma injection on different types and grades of facial wrinkles. J Cosmet Dermatol. 2017; 16(1):103–111

9
Combination Therapies

Peter W. Hashim and Gary Goldenberg

Abstract

Combination therapies involving micro-needling, platelet-rich plasma, and energy-based devices represent exciting advances in minimally invasive aesthetic medicine. With continuing efforts to maximize patient outcomes, practitioners have combined treatment modalities in order to elicit synergistic effects. Here, we examine the utility of these approaches by reviewing the relevant efficacy and safety results from studies of combination regimens.

Keywords: combination therapies, platelet-rich plasma, microneedling, laser resurfacing, drug delivery, ultrasound

Key Points

- Combination therapies capitalize on and allow for synergistic benefits from different treatment modalities.
- Platelet-rich plasma is easily combined with microneedling or laser resurfacing, leading to more effective results and shorter downtime.
- Microneedling, through its simple and rapid mechanical penetration of the stratum corneum, holds promise for transdermal delivery of drugs.
- The increased strength of combination therapies should be routinely weighed against possible increases in adverse events.

9.1 PRP with Laser Resurfacing

Platelet-rich plasma (PRP) is an autologous solution and concentrated reservoir of numerous growth factors, including platelet-derived growth factor (PDGF), vascular endothelial growth factor (VEGF), transforming growth factor (TGF), epidermal growth factor (EGF), and insulin-like growth factor (IGF).[1] Isolated from whole blood after venipuncture, PRP can be easily prepared in the office setting just prior to a planned procedure. Peripheral whole blood undergoes centrifugation to separate the desired platelet and plasma (also known as PRP) components, with a resultant 5 mL of PRP typically concentrated to contain a platelet count of at least 1,000,000/μL (note that blood draw volume, preparation techniques, and final concentration vary by system and can substantially impact the final concentration and composition; **Chapter 1**).[2] Importantly, the facility of PRP procurement and delivery allows it to be readily used in conjunction with other treatment modalities.

One important application of PRP is with laser resurfacing procedures. This combination applies the regenerative properties of PRP to the microthermal treatment zones created during resurfacing. Several studies have compared the use of laser resurfacing alone versus in combination with PRP (▶ Table 9.1).

Table 9.1 Platelet-rich plasma with laser resurfacing

Authors	Study design	N	Mean age, year (range)	Comparison	Treatment protocol	Results	Adverse effects
Shin et al. (2012)	Facial rejuvenation; control group and experimental group	22	43.7 (30–56)	1,550-nm fractional erbium glass laser + topical PRP vs. 1,550-nm fractional erbium glass laser alone	Three treatments at 4-week intervals	Non-ablative fractional laser + topical PRP led to scar improvement in 73% of patients vs. 45% with laser alone. Combination therapy also led to larger increases in collagen and fibroblasts	No long-term adverse effects
Lee et al. (2011)	Acne scars; split-face design	14	28.1 (21–38)	Fractional CO_2 laser + intradermal PRP vs. fractional CO_2 laser + intradermal NS	Two treatments at 1-month interval	CO_2 laser + intradermal PRP led to greater scar improvement and faster resolution of laser-damaged skin vs. CO_2 laser + intradermal NS	No long-term adverse effects
Na et al. (2011)	Healthy skin on the bilateral inner arms; split-body design	25	Not listed	Fractional CO_2 laser + topical PRP vs. fractional CO_2 laser + topical NS	One treatment	CO_2 laser + topical PRP led to reduced erythema and trasnspeidermal water loss in the recovery period vs. CO_2 laser + topical NS. PRP treatment was also associated with thicker collagen bundles at 1-month follow-up	No long-term adverse effect
Gawdat et al. (2014)	Acne scars; two groups, each with split-face design	30	24.8 (19–35)	Fractional CO_2 laser + topical PRP vs. fractional CO_2 laser + intradermal PRP vs. fractional CO_2 laser + intradermal NS	Three treatments at 1-month intervals	A grade of >75% improvement was seen in 67% of areas treated by CO_2 laser + intradermal PRP vs. 60% of areas treated by CO_2 laser + intradermal PRP vs. 27% of areas treated by CO_2 laser + intradermal NS. Topical PRP application yielded reduced pain vs. intradermal	PIH on the sides of two patients treated with CO_2 laser + intradermal NS

Abbreviations: PRP, platelet-rich plasma; CO_2, carbon dioxide; NS, normal saline; PIH, postinflammatory hyperpigmentation.

Shin et al[3] examined the value of dual therapy in 22 patients undergoing facial rejuvenation. Half of the patients received topical application of PRP (unspecified concentration) combined with fractional laser resurfacing, while the other half received fractional laser resurfacing alone. Subjects underwent three treatments with a non-ablative 1,550-nm fractional erbium glass laser, each separated by 4 weeks. In the combination treatment group, topical PRP was applied under occlusion for 20 minutes immediately after laser therapy. Patient-reported improvements in skin texture, elasticity, and fine wrinkles were all higher in the combination treatment group. Blinded evaluators noted clinical improvement in 73% of patients in the combination group versus 45% in the monotherapy group, although the difference between groups was not statistically significant. Biopsies performed before and 1 month after the final treatment showed that combination therapy lead to significantly greater increases in the length of the dermal–epidermal junction, the volume of collagen, and the number of fibroblasts ($p < 0.05$). There were no significant differences in adverse events between the two groups.

Lee et al[4] investigated the combination of PRP with ablative carbon dioxide (CO_2) fractional resurfacing in the treatment of acne scars. In a split-face study of 14 patients, all subjects first received full-face treatment with the fractional CO_2 laser, then intradermal injections of PRP (unspecified concentration) on one side of the face versus intradermal injections of saline on the other side. The procedure was repeated 1 month later for a total of two treatment sessions spaced 1 month apart. Results confirmed an expedited recovery time after combination therapy compared to the saline control, with the mean duration of posttreatment erythema shortened by 1.8 days, duration of edema shortened by 1 day, and the duration of crusting shortened by 0.9 days (all $p < 0.05$ between treatment groups). The investigators also graded patients' clinical improvement according to a quartile scale from 0 (no improvement) to 4 (> 75% improvement). Four months following the second treatment session, the sides of the face receiving combination therapy showed greater improvement in acne scars than the control (mean quartile improvement of 2.7 vs. 2.3; $p = 0.03$). Similarly, Na et al[5] found greater wound healing and reduced transient adverse effects when fractional CO_2 resurfacing was followed by the application of PRP. In this study, thicker collagen bundles were also noted on histological examination of PRP-treated sides relative to controls.

Expanding on such results, Gawdat et al[6] compared differential effects seen with topical versus intradermal PRP in conjunction with ablative resurfacing for management of acne scars. Thirty subjects were enrolled in the split-face study and separated into two groups. In the first group, one side of the face underwent fractional CO_2 laser resurfacing followed by intradermal injections of PRP (unspecified concentration), and the other received laser treatment followed by intradermal injections of saline. In the second group, one side of the face underwent fractional CO_2 laser resurfacing followed by intradermal injections of PRP; the other side received laser treatments followed by topical PRP application under occlusion for 15 minutes. Patients completed three sessions at monthly intervals. Results at 3 months after the final session showed that the combination of laser with PRP (regardless of whether topical or intradermal) yielded greater scar improvement than the laser control group. In addition, adverse events such as erythema, edema, and crusting resolved more quickly on the combination-treated areas. The total downtime was statistically significantly shorter in the combined topical PRP and laser group

(2.8 days) and the intradermal PRP and laser group (2.3 days) relative to the laser control group (4.4 days; $p = 0.02$). Notably, there were no significant differences between the intradermal and topical applications of PRP, with the lone exception of reduced pain scores in the topical PRP group. These findings support the notion that when used concurrently with laser resurfacing, the topical route of PRP administration allows for maximized patient comfort without compromising efficacy.

9.2 Platelet-Rich Plasma with Ultrasound

Ultrasound is another energy-based modality employed to increase the penetration of PRP. In one study of striae distensae, Suh et al[7] combined topical PRP (4.5 times concentration) with ultrasound after the application of fractional radiofrequency. Eighteen patients were treated every 2 weeks for four sessions. Two months after the final treatment, the mean width of the widest striae decreased from 0.75 to 0.27 mm. About 70% of patients reported being "very satisfied" or "extremely satisfied" with the degree of improvement. Lack of control groups receiving radiofrequency, PRP plus ultrasound, or no therapy was a major limitation to this study; however, results are encouraging and warrant further investigation, especially considering striae are a common yet challenging to treat condition.

9.3 Platelet-Rich Plasma with Microneedling

Microneedling therapy uses small gauge needles to injury deliberately and mechanically the epidermis and dermis and thereby, encourage skin rejuvenation

(▶ Fig. 9.1a–c). Puncture wounds created by microneedles promote growth factor release and wound healing cascades. Histological examinations following microneedling therapy demonstrate increases in collagen and elastic fiber formation, leading to a thicker dermis with normal-appearing architecture rather than scar-type dermal changes that occur after more extensive trauma.[8,9] The clinical applications of microneedling are wide ranging, with the largest body of literature in skin rejuvenation and the treatment of acne scars (▶ Fig. 9.2a–c and ▶ Fig. 9.3a, b) (**Chapter 6**).[10,11,12,13] In addition, there are encouraging results observed in the management of hypertrophic burn scars and melasma.[14,15,16] The possible indications for microneedling continue to expand. These investigational applications include androgenic alopecia, hyperhidrosis, striae rubra, and transdermal delivery of drugs (▶ Fig. 9.4a, b and ▶ Fig. 9.5, ▶ Fig. 9.6, ▶ Fig. 9.7, ▶ Fig. 9.8).[17,18,19,20]

Several studies have examined the differential efficacy of microneedling therapy with and without PRP (▶ Table 9.2). Using a split-face study design, Fabbrocini et al[21] compared treatment outcomes in patients with atrophic acne scars. In a study population of 12 adults, one side of each patient's face received microneedling at 1.5 mm depth plus topical PRP (4.5 times concentration), while the other only microneedling. Outcomes were examined 32 weeks after the second of two treatment sessions, spaced 8 weeks apart. Although both regimens resulted in improvements in scar severity scores, those treated with combined microneedling plus PRP demonstrated greater results (mean improvement of 47 vs. 35%; $p < 0.05$). The addition of PRP did not appear to alter posttreatment swelling or

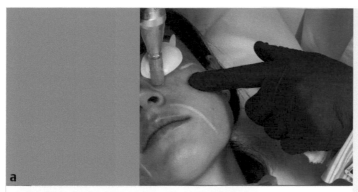

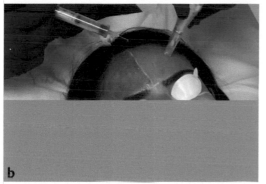

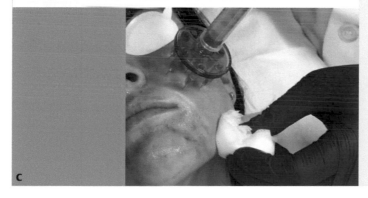

Fig. 9.1 Microneedling with PRP. (a) The microneedling device is first used to create minute puncture wounds. (b) Topical PRP is then applied to the skin using a syringe. (c) Alternatively, PRP can be injected intradermally following microneedling. (© 2017 Cutis (https://www.mdedge.com/cutis) and Gary Goldenberg.)

erythema, which were mild and common among both groups.

Asif et al[22] went a step further and evaluated the triple combination of topical PRP, intradermal PRP, and microneedling. In a split-face comparison study of 50 subjects with atrophic acne scars, half the face was treated with microneedling at 1.5 mm depth followed by intradermal injections of distilled water, and the other side with microneedling followed by intradermal injections of calcium chloride-activated PRP (5.2 times concentration) then topical PRP application. Patients completed three, monthly sessions with a final assessment performed 4 months after the last treatment. Using the Goodman's quantitative scale for acne scarring, combination microneedling and PRP led to a 62% reduction in scar severity. About 40% of these patients demonstrated an "excellent response" (two-grade improvement), while the remaining 60% had a "good response" (one-grade improvement

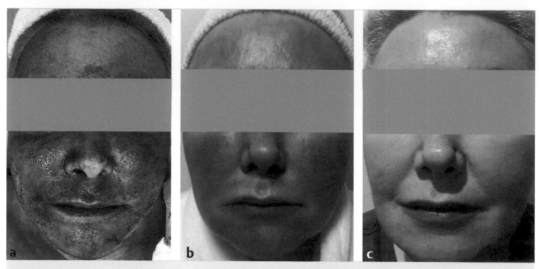

Fig. 9.2 Facial rejuvenation with microneedling and PRP, seen **(a)** immediately after treatment, **(b)** 24 hours after treatment, and **(c)** 3 days after treatment. (© Gary Goldenberg. Used with permission.)

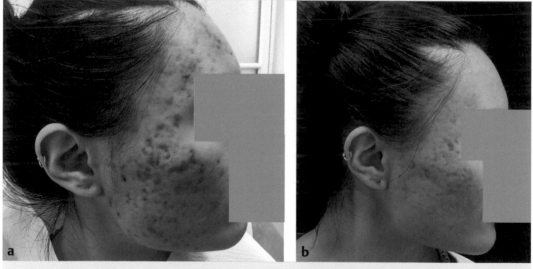

Fig. 9.3 Acne scars **(a)** before and **(b)** after treatment with microneedling and PRP. (© Gary Goldenberg. Used with permission.)

in scar severity). Importantly, no subjects failed to respond to the combination therapy. In comparison, the isolated microneedling-sterile water group also noted clinical benefits, although the effects were less dramatic. Overall scars reduced by 46% (vs. 62% with combination PRP treatment; $p < 0.00001$), with an excellent response seen in 10%, good response in 84%, and poor response in 6%. The authors noted that postprocedural erythema and skin peeling appeared to resolve slightly more quickly on the PRP-treated sides.

There is also a comparative study of microneedling at 1.5 mm depth plus PRP (4.5 times concentration) versus microneedling plus vitamin C.[23] The investigators treated 30 patients with acne scars over

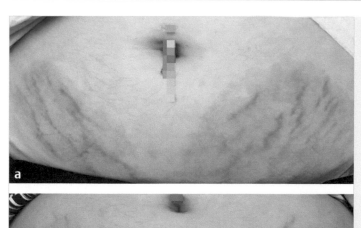

Fig. 9.4 Striae rubra. **(a)** Before and **(b)** after treatment with microneedling and PRP. (© Gary Goldenberg. Used with permission.)

4 monthly sessions in a split-faced study design. Although both treatment regimens produced clinical benefits, there was a statistically significantly higher percentage of patients who failed to demonstrate any improvement in the vitamin C group (37%) compared to the PRP group (22%; $p = 0.021$). Furthermore, 19% of PRP patients demonstrated "excellent response" (two-point improvement) but only 7% with vitamin C. The authors noted that boxcar and rolling scars tended to show better responses to treatment than ice pick scars.

9.3.1 Microneedling for Drug Delivery

Increasingly, microneedling has been examined to facilitate transdermal medication delivery. Entry of drug may occur through three possible mechanisms: (1) the creation of pores in the stratum corneum followed by the topical application of drug; (2) the coating of microneedles with drug; and/or (3) the use of hollow microneedles filled with drug, which inject directly into the skin. These varied application techniques have demonstrated utility in the delivery of numerous medications, including insulin and vaccines.[24]

Evidence suggests microneedling can increase the efficacy of photodynamic therapy (PDT). Bencini et al[25] followed 12 organ transplant patients who had previously failed classical PDT for the treatment of actinic keratosis. Patients underwent three sessions of microneedle-assisted PDT at 2-week intervals, each consisting of microneedling at 0.5 mm depth followed by the application of methylaminolevulinate under occlusion for 3 hours then finally, irradiation. All lesions showed a complete response after the three treatment sessions, with a persistent 83% clearance rate noted at the 9 month follow-up.

Enhanced delivery of topical anesthetics is another potential application of microneedling. In a study by Fabbrocini et al,[19] microneedling at the shallow depth of 0.5 mm was combined with a eutectic

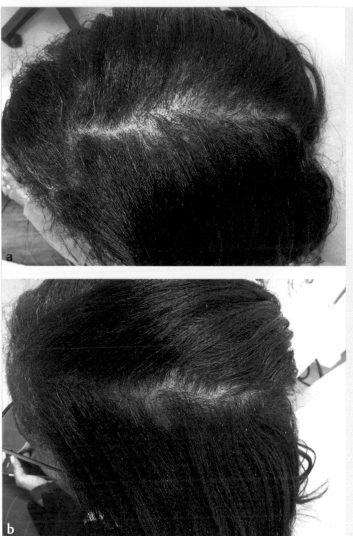

Fig. 9.5 Androgenetic alopecia. **(a)** Before and **(b)** after treatment with microneedling and PRP. (© Gary Goldenberg. Used with permission.)

mixture of lidocaine and prilocaine (EMLA). About 15 patients each received one of two treatments on the left or right forearm: on one side, topical anesthestic applied under occlusion for 60 minutes and on the other, microneedling prior to the application of topical anesthestic under occlusion for 60 minutes. Afterward, the clinicians monitored response to pain. Results found that combination treatment led to significantly lower pain scores according to the visual analog scale (51.3 vs. 20.1; $p < 0.05$). The authors reported no major side effects, with only mild erythema and swelling limited to 24 to 48 hours. It should be noted that in clinical practice, such increased absorption of anesthetic will need to be weighed against increased risk of toxicity when treating large body surface areas.

Finally, microneedling has also been shown to enhance the delivery of cosmeceutical peptides. Mohammed et al[26] used fluorescence imaging to examine the delivery of melanostatin, rigin, and pal-KTTKS on human donor skin with and without microneedling. A 2- to 22-fold signal increase was found after

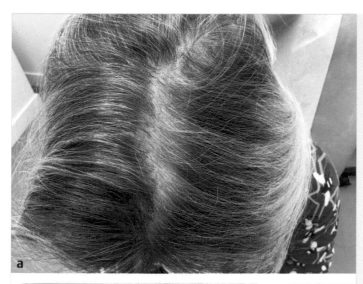
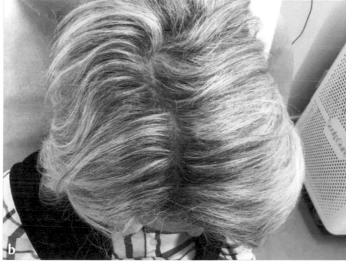

Fig. 9.6 Androgenetic alopecia. (a) Before and (b) after treatment with microneedling and PRP. (© Gary Goldenberg. Used with permission.)

microneedle-enhanced delivery of topically applied peptides, with the lowest molecular weight peptides showing the largest response to pretreatment with microneedling.

Recently, the delivery of antiwrinkle compounds through dissolving microneedle platforms has been studied.[27] About 24 women were treated for 12 weeks with dissolving microneedle patches loaded with either ascorbic acid or retinyl retinoate. Patches were applied twice daily to the periorbital crow's feet region. Wrinkle improvement was evaluated by Visiome-

ter software before and immediately after the completion of treatment. Both ascorbic acid and retinyl retinoate-loaded patches reduced skin roughness and arithmetically derived average roughness ($p < 0.001$). Importantly, there were no reports of allergic or contact dermatitis.

9.4 Microneedling with Laser Resurfacing

Less commonly, providers may combine microneedling with laser resurfacing. This combination aims to target the

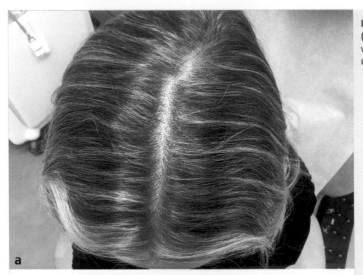
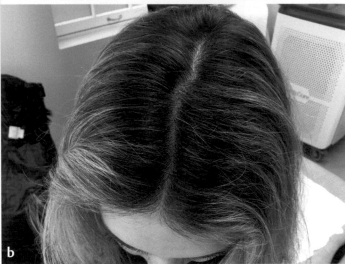

Fig. 9.7 Androgenetic alopecia. **(a)** Before and **(b)** after treatment with microneedling and PRP. (© Gary Goldenberg. Used with permission.)

epidermis and papillary dermis through laser resurfacing, while longer microneedles provide deeper penetration into the reticular dermis. It can also be considered in darker Fitzpatrick Skin types who will not tolerate more aggressive laser settings or particular wavelengths, given increased risk of adverse events. Of note, the studies to date are generally less robust and rigorously designed, so there is substantial room for ongoing investigation and protocol development.

Two studies examine the combined use of fractional radiofrequency microneedling (FRM) and laser resurfacing (▶ Table 9.3). Ryu et al[28] treated patients suffering from striae distensae according to three different protocols: FRM alone, fractional CO_2 laser alone, or combined FRM and fractional CO_2 laser. Subjects underwent three treatment sessions separated by one month. Overall, the combination group was noted to have greater clinical improvements than either single

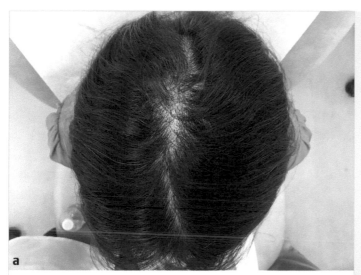
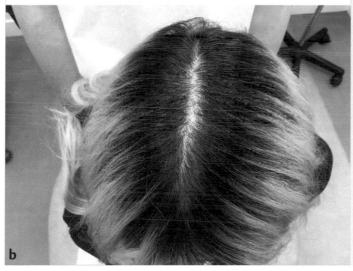

Fig. 9.8 Androgenetic alopecia. (a) Before and (b) after treatment with microneedling and PRP. (© Gary Goldenberg. Used with permission.)

modality, although comparison statistics were not provided. Biopsy specimens from before and 6 months after combination treatment demonstrated increased collagen fibers and higher expression levels of transforming growth factor-β1 in the epidermis and dermis of combination treated skin. Transient postinflammatory hyperpigmentation, pain, and pruritus were also reported more commonly in the combination group (statistical comparisons not provided).

Similarly, Fatemi Naeini et al[29] found that combined FRM and CO_2 laser therapy was more effective in treating striae alba than FRM alone, though adverse events were again increased. The combination regimen led to greater reductions in lesional surface area as well as higher patient satisfaction scores. Notably, there was a greater incidence of transient postinflammatory hyperpigmentation in combined FRM and CO_2 laser group, but all reported cases resolved within 3 months.

Table 9.2 Platelet-rich plasma with microneedling

Authors	Study design	N	Mean age, year (range)	Comparisons	Treatment protocol	Results	Adverse effects
Fabbrocini et al. (2011)	Acne scars; split-face design	12	32.2 (18–45)	Microneedling + topical PRP vs. microneedling alone	Two treatments at 8-week interval	Microneedling + PRP led to 47% improvement vs. 35% improvement with microneedling alone	No long-term adverse effects
Asif et al[22] (2016)	Acne scars; split-face design	50	25.7 (17–32)	Microneedling + topical PRP + intradermal PRP vs. microneedling + distilled water	Three treatments at 1-month intervals	Microneedling + PRP led to 62% improvement vs. 46% improvement with microneedling + distilled water	No long-term adverse effects
Chawla (2014)	Acne scars; split-face design	30	27.5 (18–34)	Microneedling + topical PRP vs. microneedling + topical vitamin C	Four treatments at 1-month intervals	Microneedling + PRP led to good or excellent response in 78% vs. 63% with microneedling + vitamin C	One patient experienced severe PIH

Abbreviations: PRP, platelet-rich plasma; PIH, postinflammatory hyperpigmentation.

Table 9.3 Fractional radiofrequency microneedling with laser resurfacing

Authors	Study design	N	Mean age, year (range)	Comparisons	Treatment protocol	Results	Adverse effects
Ryu et al. (2013)	Striae distensae; two solo therapy groups and one combination therapy group	30	30 (21–51)	Fractional CO_2 laser vs. FRM vs. fractional CO_2 laser + FRM	Three treatments at 1-month intervals	Fractional CO_2 laser + FRM combination led to greater clinical improvements than either therapy alone	PIH in 30% of patients in the combination group, with spontaneous resolution in 2 months
Fatemi Naeini et al. (2016)	Striae alba; split-body design	48 pairs of striae from 6 patients	30.2 (no range listed)	FMR vs. FMR + fractional CO_2 laser	FMR group: three treatments at 4-week intervals; FMR + laser group: five treatments at 4-week intervals (one treatment with laser, then three treatments with FMR, and finally one treatment with FMR + laser)	Fractional CO_2 laser + FRM combination led to 75% improvement vs. 50% improvement in the FMR group	PIH in 19% of patients in the combination group, with spontaneous resolution in 3 months

Abbreviations: FRM, fractional radiofrequency microneedling; PIH, postinflammatory hyperpigmentation.

9.5 Conclusion

Combination therapies offer clinicians a wide array of treatment options. PRP continues to gain popularity as an adjunctive agent in dermatologic and plastic surgery procedures, with a growing body of literature demonstrating utility in augmenting the effects of microneedling and laser therapy. Other combination procedures have been shown to boost efficacy as well, although the evidence is considerably weaker at this time and consideration must be given to possible increases in adverse events. Further research into the ideal protocols to achieve maximal efficacy and safety are necessary. We anticipate continued advances in the technology and delivery systems intended to optimize outcomes and shorten recovery.

References

[1] Lubkowska A, Dolegowska B, Banfi G. Growth factor content in PRP and their applicability in medicine. J Biol Regul Homeost Agents. 2012; 26(2) Suppl 1:3S–22S

[2] Marx RE. Platelet-rich plasma (PRP): what is PRP and what is not PRP? Implant Dent. 2001; 10(4):225–228

[3] Shin MK, Lee JH, Lee SJ, Kim NI. Platelet-rich plasma combined with fractional laser therapy for skin rejuvenation. Dermatol Surg. 2012; 38(4):623–630

[4] Lee JW, Kim BJ, Kim MN, Mun SK. The efficacy of autologous platelet rich plasma combined with ablative carbon dioxide fractional resurfacing for acne scars: a simultaneous split-face trial. Dermatol Surg. 2011; 37(7):931–938

[5] Na JI, Choi JW, Choi HR, et al. Rapid healing and reduced erythema after ablative fractional carbon dioxide laser resurfacing combined with the application of autologous platelet-rich plasma. Dermatol Surg. 2011; 37(4):463–468

[6] Gawdat HI, Hegazy RA, Fawzy MM, Fathy M. Autologous platelet rich plasma: topical versus intradermal after fractional ablative carbon dioxide laser treatment of atrophic acne scars. Dermatol Surg. 2014; 40(2):152–161

[7] Suh DH, Lee SJ, Lee JH, Kim HJ, Shin MK, Song KY. Treatment of striae distensae combined enhanced penetration platelet-rich plasma and ultrasound after plasma fractional radiofrequency. J Cosmet Laser Ther. 2012; 14(6):272–276

[8] Aust MC, Fernandes D, Kolokythas P, Kaplan HM, Vogt PM. Percutaneous collagen induction therapy: an alternative treatment for scars, wrinkles, and skin laxity. Plast Reconstr Surg. 2008; 121(4):1421–1429

[9] Schwarz M, Laaff H. A prospective controlled assessment of microneedling with the Dermaroller device. Plast Reconstr Surg. 2011; 127(6):146e–148e

[10] El-Domyati M, Barakat M, Awad S, Medhat W, El-Fakahany H, Farag H. Microneedling therapy for atrophic acne scars: an objective evaluation. J Clin Aesthet Dermatol. 2015; 8(7):36–42

[11] Leheta T, El Tawdy A, Abdel Hay R, Farid S. Percutaneous collagen induction versus full-concentration trichloroacetic acid in the treatment of atrophic acne scars. Dermatol Surg. 2011; 37(2):207–216

[12] Fabbrocini G, De Vita V, Pastore F, et al. Collagen induction therapy for the treatment of upper lip wrinkles. J Dermatolog Treat. 2012; 23(2):144–152

[13] Leheta TM, Abdel Hay RM, El Garem YF. Deep peeling using phenol versus percutaneous collagen induction combined with trichloroacetic acid 20% in atrophic post-acne scars: a randomized controlled trial. J Dermatolog Treat. 2014; 25(2):130–136

[14] Aust MC, Knobloch K, Reimers K, et al. Percutaneous collagen induction therapy: an alternative treatment for burn scars. Burns. 2010; 36(6):836–843

[15] Fabbrocini G, De Vita V, Fardella N, et al. Skin needling to enhance depigmenting serum penetration in the treatment of melasma. Plast Surg Int. 2011; 2011:158:241

[16] Cho SB, Lee SJ, Kang JM, Kim YK, Kim TY, Kim DH. The treatment of burn scar-induced contracture with the pinhole method and collagen induction therapy: a case report. J Eur Acad Dermatol Venereol. 2008; 22(4):513–514

[17] Dhurat R, Mathapati S. Response to microneedling treatment in men with androgenetic alopecia who failed to respond to conventional therapy. Indian J Dermatol. 2015; 60(3):260–263

[18] Dhurat R, Sukesh M, Avhad G, Dandale A, Pal A, Pund P. A randomized evaluator blinded study of effect of microneedling in androgenetic alopecia: a pilot study. Int J Trichology. 2013; 5(1):6–11

[19] Fabbrocini G, De Vita V, Izzo R, Monfrecola G. The use of skin needling for the delivery of a eutectic mixture of local anesthetics. G Ital Dermatol Venereol. 2014; 149(5):581–585

[20] Kim M, Shin JY, Lee J, Kim JY, Oh SH. Efficacy of fractional microneedle radiofrequency device in the treatment of primary axillary hyperhidrosis: a pilot study. Dermatology. 2013; 227(3):243–249

[21] Fabbrocini G, De Vita V, Pastore F, et al. Combined use of skin needling and platelet-rich plasma in acne scarring treatment. Cosmetic Dermatology. 2011; 24(4):177–183

[22] Asif M, Kanodia S, Singh K. Combined autologous platelet-rich plasma with microneedling verses microneedling with distilled water in the treatment of atrophic acne scars: a concurrent split-face study. J Cosmet Dermatol. 2016; 15(4):434–443

[23] Chawla S. Split face comparative study of microneedling with PRP versus microneedling with vitamin C in treating atrophic post acne scars. J Cutan Aesthet Surg. 2014; 7(4):209–212

[24] Cheung K, Das DB. Microneedles for drug delivery: trends and progress. Drug Deliv. 2016; 23(7):2338–2354

[25] Bencini PL, Galimberti MG, Pellacani G, Longo C. Application of photodynamic therapy combined with pre-illumination microneedling in the treatment of actinic keratosis in organ transplant recipients. Br J Dermatol. 2012; 167(5):1193–1194

[26] Mohammed YH, Yamada M, Lin LL, et al. Microneedle enhanced delivery of cosmeceutically relevant peptides in human skin. PLoS One. 2014; 9(7):e101956

[27] Kim M, Yang H, Kim H, Jung H, Jung H. Novel cosmetic patches for wrinkle improvement: retinyl retinoate- and ascorbic acid-loaded dissolving microneedles. Int J Cosmet Sci. 2014; 36(3):207–212

[28] Ryu HW, Kim SA, Jung HR, Ryoo YW, Lee KS, Cho JW. Clinical improvement of striae distensae in Korean patients using a combination of fractionated microneedle radiofrequency and fractional carbon dioxide laser. Dermatol Surg. 2013; 39(10): 1452–1458

[29] Fatemi Naeini F, Behfar S, Abtahi-Naeini B, Keyvan S, Pourazizi M. Promising option for treatment of striae alba: fractionated microneedle radiofrequency in combination with fractional carbon dioxide laser. Dermatol Res Pract. 2016; 2016:2896345

10

Complications Associated with PRP and Microneedling in Aesthetic Medicine

Tatjana Pavicic and Matthias Aust

Abstract

Microneedling and platelet-rich plasma are two minimally invasive, office-based procedures for rejuvenation, resurfacing, wound healing, and hair restoration with long-lasting effects and minimal downtime. Treatments are performed at approximately 4-week intervals. Patients should be educated on the anticipated outcomes, delayed time to response, and need for multiple sittings. The main contraindication for both procedures is active skin infection in the area targeted for therapy. History of keloidal or hypertrophic scars should also be considered, particularly prior to microneedling. There are usually no or few post-treatment sequelae with the exception of mild bruising, erythema, edema and skin peeling, which typically resolve in 2 to 3 days, depending on intensity. More severe adverse events are rare and generally limited to hypersensitivity reactions or infection. Detailed history of any prior allergic reactions or recent infections and use of strict aseptic techniques allow the provider to mostly avoid these unwanted effects. For each adverse event, this chapter will provide background as well as advice on avoidance and treatment. With a thorough understanding of the expected adverse events, the aesthetic practitioner can optimize outcomes and ensure satisfied patients.

Keywords: facial rejuvenation, microneedling, neocollagenesis, percutaneous collagen induction, platelet-rich plasma

Key Points

- Microneedling and platelet-rich plasma (PRP) are effective treatments for fine lines, wrinkles, acne or other scarring, stretch marks, melasma or hyperpigmention, and alopecia and can be used on any skin type.
- Microneedling and injection of PRP are medical treatments that break the outer layer of the skin and strict aseptic technique must be practiced.
- Needle length should be appropriate for the treatment indication, anatomic location, and skin quality to avoid unnecessary trauma and ensure optimal outcomes.
- All topical products applied before, during, and/or immediately after microneedling must be sterile and non-allergenic to minimize dermal absorption of products that may trigger an inflammatory or foreign body response.

10.1 Introduction

Skin condition is an important determinant of human attractiveness,[1] but with age and increased exposure to ultraviolet radiation and other lifestyle factors such as poor nutrition, alcohol consumption, and smoking, the complexion is subject to a number of undesirable changes including dryness, roughness, development of surface blood vessels, uneven pigmentation, loss of elasticity, and wrinkling. In younger patients, atrophic scarring commonly as a complication of acne vulgaris can have a significant effect on self-esteem and quality of life.[2]

A number of minimally invasive skin rejuvenation and resurfacing procedures are available to correct or ameliorate these changes, such as ablative and nonablative lasers, radiofrequency, ultrasound, chemical peels, dermabrasion, injectable fillers, and microneedling. All are designed to create dermal injury and thereby, stimulate wound repair and neocollagenesis, but differ in the type of injury utilized. Microneedling, or collagen induction therapy, is one such technique that uses fine needles to puncture the skin at various depths and create controlled skin injury without damaging the full epidermis (▶ Fig. 10.1).[3] Each puncture creates a channel in the dermis, triggering the release of growth factors and cytokines.[4,5] These, in turn, stimulate neocollagenesis,

neoelastogenesis, and angiogenesis. A number of microneedling devices are available such as dermal rollers and the more recently developed, dermal stamps or automated pens.[6] Microneedling is safe on any skin type due to the lack of thermal energy and is an effective technique for the treatment of fine lines, wrinkles, loose skin, acne or other scarring, stretch marks, and potentially melasma or hyperpigmentation as well as alopecia. Combining it with other topical products, such as growth factors, vitamin A and/or C, and more recently, platelet-rich plasma (PRP), may enhance drug delivery and overall benefits. It is hypothesized that the additional growth factors and cytokines from the PRP act synergistically with the already accelerated neocollagenesis from microneedling for even more rapid and robust collagen remodeling. This chapter will review the techniques for optimal results and complication avoidance with microneedling and PRP.

10.2 Patient Suitability

Both microneedling and PRP are suitable for all skin types, even darker Fitzpatrick tones with minimal risk of inducing hypopigmentation.[4,7] Contraindications are primarily disease related. For microneedling, care must be taken not to treat patients with any active infections or

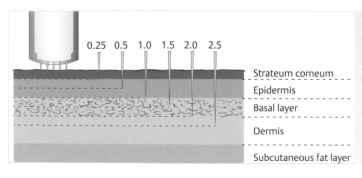

Fig. 10.1 Needle length (mm) and skin structure targeted. Note: True depth of penetration depends on anatomic location.

0.25 0.5 1.0 1.5 2.0 2.5

Strateum corneum

Epidermis

Basal layer

Dermis

Subcutaneous fat layer

conditions that may be spread or exacerbated by skin puncture (i.e., pathergy). History of keloidal or hypertrophic scars may also limit therapy, particularly at certain anatomic locations.

Contraindications for PRP include metastatic or systemic diseases that prevent the patient's blood from being used for therapy; low platelet or fibrinogen counts; anemia; infections in the therapy areas; and heavy nicotine and alcohol consumption. Corticosteroid injections and nonsteroidal anti-inflammatory drugs should be avoided if possible, as they may prevent the inflammation that is essential for the PRP serum to work. In addition, anticoagulant prescription medications or antiplatelet therapy should be stopped for a few weeks before and after PRP therapy. Certain chemotherapy agents such as tamoxifen alter platelet function and thus should also be taken into consideration when designing an optimal treatment plan, though the true effects on outcomes is unknown at this time.

10.3 Pre- and Postprocedure Care

A careful patient history should be taken to obtain information on any allergic reactions, in particular reactions to the topical treatments that will be used before and after therapy and to metals that may be present in the microneedles such as nickel, silver, or gold. Data suggest that at least 1 month prior to treatment, patients should begin applying vitamins A and C formulations twice-daily to the target area to maximize dermal collagen formation.[7] Vitamin A influences numerous genes that control the proliferation and differentiation of epidermal and dermal cells, while vitamin C is essential for normal collagen production.[7]

The treatment area should be cleansed fully of makeup or other debris then anesthetized with topical anesthetic for 45 minutes to 1 hour, during which time the PRP can be prepared. Immediately prior to treatment, the skin is disinfected again with normal saline and 70% ethanol to remove all anesthetic. The skin should be wiped with sterile saline pads/gauze after the session. During combination treatments, some providers leave PRP on the surface of the skin for up to 24 hours to allow for full platelet degranulation. Cold compresses can be applied to reduce swelling. Application of nonapproved topical products prior to, during, and after microneedling can introduce immunogenic particles into the dermis and cause hypersensitivity reactions, so should be avoided. Space treatments by approximately 4 weeks duration, and patients should be advised that the full cycle of collagen synthesis and remodeling is a slow, multistage process that can take up to 10 to 12 months, so improvement will likely not be evident during their first sessions.[4] It is important to adhere to the schedule and not discontinue after one or two sessions; photos of the skin before and after microneedling treatments will help patients judge their progress. Diligent sun protection and sunscreen is paramount. Patients can generally return to work the next day, but should avoid applying makeup or other topical agents (other than those provided) for the first 24 hours while the needling channels reseal.

10.4 Adverse Events: Avoidance and Treatment

The rate of adverse events associated with microneedling and PRP is low and the majority mild as a result of trauma from needles piercing the skin (▶ Fig. 10.2, ▶ Fig. 10.3, ▶ Fig. 10.4, ▶ Fig. 10.5). Small-scale studies evaluating the effects of microneedling with and without the application of PRP,

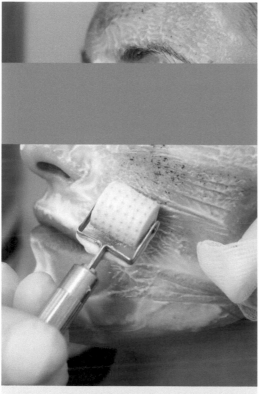

Fig. 10.2 Patient immediately after microneedling to a depth of 1 mm illustrating erythema and pinpoint bleeding.

most often for the treatment of atrophic scars, have shown that patients tend to experience 2 to 3 days of mild bruising, erythema, edema, and peeling after treatment regardless of the addition of PRP.[8,9, 10,11,12] Skin may also feel warm, tight, and pruritic for a short while (much like an ultraviolet burn), but this sensation normally resolves in 12 to 48 hours.

10.4.1 Bruising/Petechiae

It is important to select the correct length of microneedle for the required indication, bearing in mind that skin thickness varies at different parts of the face and body as well as from individual to individual. Deeper depth treatments may be associated with more bruising and pinpoint bleeding immediately postprocedure (▶ Fig. 10.2, ▶ Fig. 10.3, ▶ Fig. 10.4a, b). In order to avoid excessive bruising and hematoma after PRP treatment, a needle size in the range 30 to 32 gauge should be selected and no larger than 27 gauge. Bruising typically takes the form of many sporadic or clustered petechiae, resembling coffee grounds or cayenne pepper. This bruising will resolve spontaneously over 2 to 5 days but may potentially be treated with cold compresses, vitamin K cream, arnica gel, and even certain laser

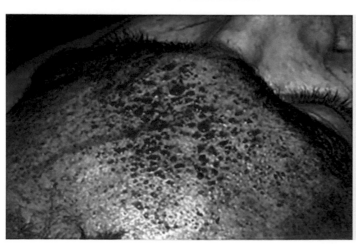

Fig. 10.3 Patient immediately after microneedling to a depth of 3 mm.

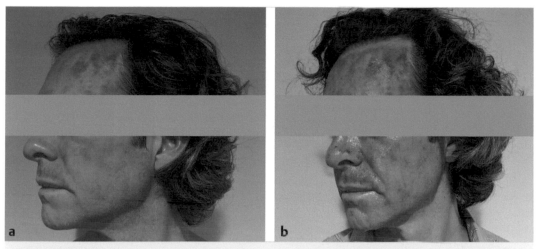

Fig. 10.4 (a, b) Patient at days 1 and 2 post-microneedling with topical platelet-rich plasma.

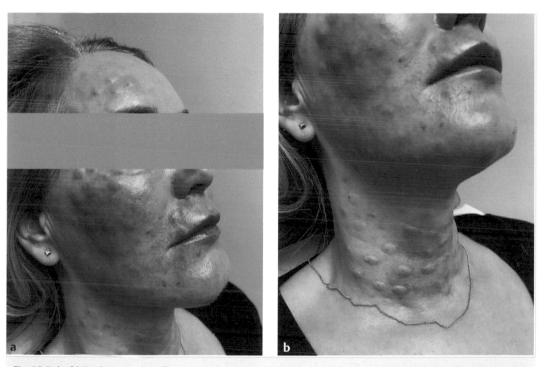

Fig. 10.5 (a, b) Erythema and swelling in a patient immediately after receiving injections of platelet-rich plasma with a 30-gauge needle.

therapies (i.e., pulse dye laser). A number of steps can be taken to minimize bruising: avoiding all blood-thinning medications or supplements starting 1 week prior to the procedure, limiting vigorous exercise for the first 24 hours to prevent elevated blood pressure, and staying out of the sun while bruising persists.

10.4.2 Erythema

Immediately after treatment, skin redness is normal and should resolve in approximately 2 to 3 days (▶ Fig. 10.4a, b). Some patients experience prolonged erythema (2 to 3 weeks) that may resemble hyperpigmentation with dark-colored spots, due to iron deposition from the subcutaneous blood (hemosiderosis). Microneedling stimulates angiogenesis by increasing levels of vascular endothelial growth factor, and this may be the cause of the prolonged erythema observed in some patients. Those with rosacea have a higher risk of developing postinjection or needling erythema and should be warned of this possibility. Evidence suggests that vitamin K cream is useful in accelerating resolution of erythema.[13]

10.4.3 Edema

Transient swelling immediately after the procedure is normal and related to cutaneous trauma. The majority of cases are mild and these dissipate within 1 to 3 days. Treatment and avoidance techniques are as for bruising.

10.4.4 Desquamation

It is normal for the skin to feel xerotic and grainy or to peel within the few days after microneedling treatments. Microneedling creates a large number of tiny puncture wounds with production of a new epidermal layer and shedding of the old. This desquamation is minimal, similar to a mild sunburn, and usually subsides within a week.

10.4.5 Skin Marking

When performing microneedling with dermal rollers, care must be taken to avoid the so-called "tram track" effect.[14] These regular, parallel lines are thought to occur when the roller head is not lifted from the skin before the next pass, hence it moves back and forth with needles repeatedly piercing skin in the same area. The effect is more likely to occur when passing over bony prominences such as the temporal area, zygomatic arch, and forehead. When treating these areas, needle depth should be limited to less than 2.0 mm (3.0 mm in hands of experienced practitioners depending on skin thickness) and strong pressure should be avoided.[4] In addition, the roller should be lifted after each pass, and repositioned a few millimeters away from the previous starting point.

10.4.6 Hyperpigmentation

Increased pigmentation was reported in a single case report in which PRP was applied over previously existing pigmented skin lesions.[15] Thus, the authors advise that PRP should not be used to attenuate postinflammatory hyperpigmentation (PIH) (i.e., after laser treatment) or on facial areas with preexisting hyperpigmentation. Topical skin bleaching agents such as vitamin C, tranexamic acid, kojic acid, or hydroquinone may help the resolution of this rare PRP-related PIH.

Microneedling may also rarely be associated with hyperpigmentation. Discoloration is more likely to occur if the needle depth is 1.5 mm or deeper, and the procedure is performed too frequently. In these situations, excessive irritation to the skin can lead to PIH. Hence, microneedling procedures should be spaced 4 to 6 weeks apart. If hyperpigmentation does occur, the procedure should not be repeated at that time. In darker skin types, the bleaching agents highlighted above may be used to pretreat the skin in order to reduce the activity of melanocytes and even the keratinocyte layer (in a similar manner to medium depth skin peels), as well as between treatment sessions after the skin has healed completely. Long-lasting hyperpigmentation after microneedling does not occur. The procedure has been associated with a decrease in levels of melanocyte-stimulating hormone and upregulation of interleukin-10 with no effect on skin melanocytes.[16]

10.4.7 Hypersensitivity Reactions

Although uncommon, some patients may develop hypersensitivity reactions to products applied at the time of microneedling or because of a reaction to the needles themselves. The duration of time that microchannels remain open depends on the diameter and length of the needle. While the external-most surface of the skin may be restored in the first few hours, the full channel depth is thought to remain open for at least 8 hours and possibly up to 24. In addition to aseptic procedure techniques, care must, therefore, be taken to ensure that all topical products used during and/or immediately after microneedling are sterile, formulated for use on broken skin, and only contain pure ingredients to minimize dermal absorption of products that may trigger an inflammatory or foreign body response. Many topical formulations are intended to be applied *onto* not *into* the skin.

Facial hypersensitivity reactions have been associated with the application of products before microneedle therapy. In one report, researchers studied three women who developed facial granulomas after receiving microneedle therapy for skin rejuvenation.[17] Biopsy results showed foreign body-type granulomas, and tissue culture results were negative.[17] Two of the three patients had received microinjection of the same lipophilic vitamin C topical moisturizer and patch tested positively to the product. The third patient, who was treated with different topical products during three sessions of microneedle therapy, refused a patch test 3 months after her final session. Clinical skin examination revealed erythematosus papules on the bilateral cheeks and chin. In cases such as these, initial treatment is with intralesional corticosteroids. However, prolonged courses of anti-inflammatory or immunomodulator medications may be required.

Two case reports documented nickel hypersensitivity reactions in patients treated with nickle-containing microneedles. In the first, a 24-year-old woman who received treatment for post-acne atrophic facial scars developed erythmatous papules along the lines of the microneedling.[18] She did not develop any systemic symptoms and responded to a short course of oral prednisolone followed by mild topical corticosteroids. Subsequent patch testing confirmed an allergy to nickel sulfate. In the second report, two sisters aged 34 and 44 years underwent facial skin needling by a trained practitioner.[19] Both developed marked neck lymphadenopathy within 24 hours. Moreover, the older sibling experienced immediate intense localized erythema with further deterioration in the subsequent 2 weeks, developing an erythmatous papular rash on the face, trunk, and limbs. Hospitalization with oral and topical corticosteroid treatment led to gradual improvement over 2 weeks. Patch testing showed a reaction to nickel sulfate. The manufacturer confirmed that the roller needles contained up to 0.006% sulfur and 0.8% nickel bound to surgical-grade stainless steel alloy.

10.4.8 Infection

Since micropores close soon after needling, postprocedure infections are rare; however, as with any procedure that pierces the epidermis, there is a risk of introducing pathogens into the skin. If treatment targets the perioral area and the individual has a history of herpes simplex, prophylactic therapy with valaciclovir (500 mg twice-daily for 3–5 days or equivalent regimen) can be started before treatment to reduce the likelihood of outbreak. If the patient has not received prophylaxis, abortive therapy with valaciclovir at a dose of 2 g twice-daily should be given at the first signs or symptoms.

A recent case report described an unusual presentation of *Tinea corporis* that emerged simultaneously on both arms and legs in a 26-year-old woman.[20] The lesions corresponded with sites where the woman had been using a home, 0.5 mm microneedling roller during the 3 weeks prior to the appearance of the lesions. The patient reported cleaning her skin and the device before and after use with 70% ethanol. A cutaneous biopsy confirmed *Microsporum canis* infection, and the patient's cat was later confirmed as the source.

To avoid contamination during microneedling, strict sterile and/or clean technique is recommended, including prepping the treatment sites with an effective topical disinfectant, carefully removing the needle and syringe from sterile packaging, wearing gloves throughout the procedure, and ensuring that the needle is not contaminated during the procedure.

PRP treatment, in contrast, uses the patient's own blood, so there is minimal risk of a transmissible infection and allergic reaction. Labeling meticulously each patient's whole blood and resultant plasma is critical, as inadvertent mix-up of vials or syringes is one of the few ways that blood-borne infection or severe systemic hypersensitivity reaction (i.e., blood type mismatch) can occur. Taking standard sharps precautions helps protect providers against needle sticks.

10.5 Conclusion

As the demand for nonsurgical or minimally invasive procedures to combat the visible signs of aging or to improve scarred and blemished tissue continues to rise, so does the popularity of regenerative treatments such as microneedling and PRP. Though the medical literature evaluating microneedling with and without PRP is nascent and has limitations, available evidence suggests that both techniques are effective for a variety of aesthetic indications and their use in combination may improve cosmetic outcomes with no increase in adverse events. These procedures are extremely well tolerated with minimal adverse events if performed under strict aseptic and/or clean conditions and if the PRP kits and microneedling devices are used according to manufacturers' guidelines. Transient trauma-related reactions are expected and self-limited. Postinflammatory erythema and/or hyperpigmentation may occur, but are less likely than after energy-based treatments.

References

[1] Samson N, Fink B, Matts P. Interaction of skin color distribution and skin surface topography cues in the perception of female facial age and health. J Cosmet Dermatol. 2011; 10(1): 78–84
[2] Gozali MV, Zhou B. Effective treatments of atrophic acne scars. J Clin Aesthet Dermatol. 2015; 8(5):33–40
[3] Alster TS, Graham PM. Microneedling: a review and practical guide. Dermatol Surg. 2018; 44(3):397–404
[4] Aust MC, Fernandes D, Kolokythas P, Kaplan HM, Vogt PM. Percutaneous collagen induction therapy: an alternative

treatment for scars, wrinkles, and skin laxity. Plast Reconstr Surg. 2008; 121(4):1421–1429

[5] Fernandes D, Signorini M. Combating photoaging with percutaneous collagen induction. Clin Dermatol. 2008; 26(2): 192–199

[6] Singh A, Yadav S. Microneedling: advances and widening horizons. Indian Dermatol Online J. 2016; 7(4):244–254

[7] Aust MC, Knobloch K, Reimers K, et al. Percutaneous collagen induction therapy: an alternative treatment for burn scars. Burns. 2010; 36(6):836–843

[8] Asif M, Kanodia S, Singh K. Combined autologous platelet-rich plasma with microneedling verses microneedling with distilled water in the treatment of atrophic acne scars: a concurrent split-face study. J Cosmet Dermatol. 2016; 15(4): 434–443

[9] Chawla S. Split face comparative study of microneedling with PRP versus microneedling with vitamin C in treating atrophic post acne scars. J Cutan Aesthet Surg. 2014; 7(4):209–212

[10] Hashim PW, Levy Z, Cohen JL, Goldenberg G. Microneedling therapy with and without platelet-rich plasma. Cutis. 2017; 99(4):239–242

[11] Fabbrocini G, De Vita V, Pastore F, et al. Combined use of skin needling and platelet-rich plasma in acne scarring treatment. Cosmet Dermatol. 2011; 24(4):177–183

[12] Yaseen U, Shah S, Bashir A. Combination of platelet rich plasma and microneedling in the management of atrophic acne scars. Int J Res Dermatol. 2017; 3(3):346–350

[13] Cohen JL, Bhatia AC. The role of topical vitamin K oxide gel in the resolution of postprocedural purpura. J Drugs Dermatol. 2009; 8(11):1020–1024

[14] Pahwa M, Pahwa P, Zaheer A. "Tram track effect" after treatment of acne scars using a microneedling device. Dermatol Surg. 2012; 38(7 Pt 1):1107–1108

[15] Uysal CA, Ertas NM. Platelet-rich plasma increases pigmentation. J Craniofac Surg. 2017; 28(8):e793

[16] Aust MC, Reimers K, Repenning C, et al. Percutaneous collagen induction: minimally invasive skin rejuvenation without risk of hyperpigmentation-fact or fiction? Plast Reconstr Surg. 2008; 122(5):1553–1563

[17] Soltani-Arabshahi R, Wong JW, Duffy KL, Powell DL. Facial allergic granulomatous reaction and systemic hypersensitivity associated with microneedle therapy for skin rejuvenation. JAMA Dermatol. 2014; 150(1):68–72

[18] Yadav S, Dogra S. A cutaneous reaction to microneedling for post-acne scarring caused by nickel hypersensitivity. Aesthet Surg J. 2016; 36(4):NP168–NP170

[19] Pratsou P, Gach J. Severe systemic reaction associated with skin microneedling therapy in 2 sisters: a previously unrecognized potential for complications? J Am Acad Dermatol. 2013; 68 4, Supple 1:AB219, Abstract P6998

[20] da Cunha NMM, Campos SLA, Fidalgo AIPC. Unusual presentation of Tinea Corporis associated with the use of a microneedling device. Aesthet Surg J. 2017; 37(7):NP69–NP72

Index